NEOLIBERAL HEALTH ORGANIZING

Critical Cultural Studies in Global Health Communication

Global changes in migratory patterns, the increasing health inequalities faced by the poor, the health risks faced by communities at the margins of global societies, and the communicative nature of health problems have drawn additional attention to the relevance of studying health communication processes across global cultures. This series will challenge West-centric ideals of health and human behavior by publishing theoretically provacative, pedagogically critical volumes addressing the intersection of communication principles and practices with health concepts and structures. The intent of the Series is foregrounding knowledge that creates openings for transforming structures of injustice and exploitation underlying global health inequalities. Manuscript progrposales should be addressed to Series Co-editor Mohan J. Dutta at cnmhead@nus.edu.sg

Series Titles

Volume 1 *Prescribing HIV Prevention: Bringing Culture into Global Health Communication*, Nicola Bulled
Volume 2 *Neoliberal Health Organizing: Communication, Meaning, and Politics*, Mohan J. Dutta

Neoliberal Health Organizing

Communication, Meaning, and Politics

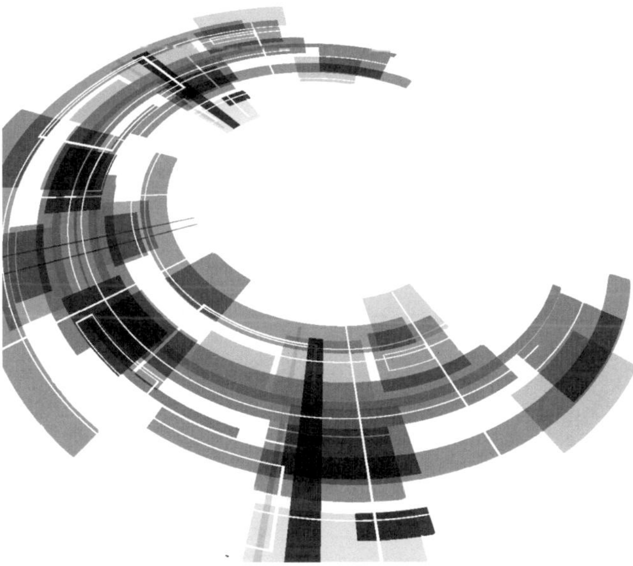

Mohan J. Dutta

Routledge
Taylor & Francis Group
LONDON AND NEW YORK

First published 2015 by Left Coast Press, Inc.

Published 2016 by Routledge
2 Park Square, Milton Park, Abingdon, Oxon OX14 4RN
711 Third Avenue, New York, NY 10017, USA

Routledge is an imprint of the Taylor & Francis Group, an informa business

Library of Congress Cataloging-in-Publication Data
Dutta, Mohan J., author.
Neoliberal health organizing : communication, meaning, and politics / Mohan Dutta.
p. ; cm. — (Critical cultural studies in global health communication ; volume 2)
Includes bibliographical references and index.
ISBN 978-1-62958-048-7 (hardcover : alk. paper) — ISBN 978-1-62958-049-4 (paperback : alk. paper) — ISBN 978-1-62958-050-0 (institutional eBook) — ISBN 978-1-62958-051-7 (consumer eBook)
I. Title. II. Series: Critical cultural studies in global health communication ; v. 2.
[DNLM: 1. Global Health. 2. Health Services—economics. 3. Politics. WA 530.1]
RA418
362.1—dc23
2014048987

ISBN 978-1-62958-049-4 paperback
ISBN 978-1-62958-048-7 hardcover

CONTENTS

For
Trisha and Shloke

ACKNOWLEDGMENTS

In June 2012, our family moved to Singapore. A new environment, with new challenges and opportunities awaited us. Our move to Singapore marked a number of choices we made, including wanting to be closer to our parents, siblings, and extended families in India, and wanting to participate in an emerging conversation on Asian modernities amid the shifting landscape of global political and economic structures. With an aging extended family with many health care needs, being in Singapore enabled us to participate in the networks of care that we grew up amid, an opportunity to give back to the uncles and aunts who now had to negotiate the challenges of seeking health care.

This book thus owes a great deal to this transitioning process and to all those that enabled the transition. Millie Rivera opened me up to this possibility of the emerging Asian century, and I am grateful to her for creating an invitational space in the Department of Communications and New Media (CNM) at the National University of Singapore (NUS). CNM is an amazing space, filled with laughter and camaraderie, and nourished by a whole lot of nurturing and intellectual curiosity. Meditation, pranks, and love for each other are integral to the CNM life, and I continue to learn a great deal from this amazing department of smart and loving colleagues. The opportunities I had in exchanging thoughts with CNM colleagues T. T. Sreekumar, Weiyu Zhang, Iccha Basnyat, Lonce Wyse, and Ingrid Hoofd invited me to consider new possibilities, challenged my own thinking, and inspired my imagination. At NUS, Prasenjit Duara, Brenda Yeoh, and Chua Beng Huat offered inspiration through their work and through conversations.

My current and former colleagues at Purdue William Collins, Josh Boyd, Howard Sypher, Glenn Sparks, Beverly Davenport, Patrice Buzanell, Robin Clair, Steve Wilson, Jeong Nam Kim, Lorraine Kisselburgh, Charles Stewart, and Stacey Connaughton, will always hold a special place in my heart for their camaraderie and for the intellectual conversations they have offered over the last decade. I owe a great deal to the intellectual inspirations offered by Raka Shome, Devika Chawla, Tom Nakayama, Soyini Madison, Heather Zoller, Phaedra Pezzullo, Dana Cloud, Jan Servaes, Karin Wilkins, Rafael Obregon, Nick Couldry, Shiv Ganesh, Srivi

Ramasubramaniam, George Cheney, Maite Soto, Arvind Singhal, and Gary Kreps. The lessons offered by Collin Airhihenbuwa, Charles Briggs, Clara Mantini Briggs, Amartya Sen, Nicola Bulled, Arturo Escobar, William Robinson, Joseph Stiglitz, Elinor Ostrum, Vicente Navarro, Howard Waitzkin, David Harvey, and Deborah Lupton fostered possibilities for understanding the relationship of communication to the broader social and structural contexts that constitute health. In health communication, Teri Thompson, Gary Kreps, Barbara Sharf, Laura Ellingson, Lynn Harter, David Novak, Jeff Peterson, and Elaine Hsieh offered much inspiration through their own work and support.

I have always felt that my students have been integral to the development of my intellectual trajectory, my empirical work, and my direction as an activist. Debalina Mookerjee, Rebecca DeSouza, Ambar Basu, Mahuya Pal, Iccha Basnyat, and Induk Kim participated as sojourners in some of my earliest adventures into theorizing. Shaunak Sastry, Sydney Dillard, Rati Kumar, Agaptus Anaele, Uttaran Dutta, and Christina Jones worked as collaborators in solidarity in one of the first large-scale implementation projects grounded in the culture-centered approach in Lake and Marion Counties of Indiana. My students at the Center for Culture-Centered Approach to Research and Evaluation (CARE) at NUS, Satveer Kaur, Sarah Comer, Abdul Rahman, Naomi Tan, Ahmed Abid, and Julio Etchart are partners in our community-activist collaborations, seeking to map out spaces of social change. Postdoctoral researchers at CARE, Jagadish Thaker, Kang Sun, Asha Pandi, Arnab Chowdhury, and Dyah Pitaloka are vital collaborators on our ongoing projects of social change. A special thanks to Asha Pandi for her diligent support in putting together the index for this book.

My friends in the activist community, Samarendra Das, Delowar Jahan, P. Satheesh, Peck Hoon, and Vanessa and Jolovan Wham are everyday inspirations for communication for social change. They embody the spirit of commitment in the face of challenges and structural constraints. Their optimism, modeled through their participation in processes of social change, guide my own theoretical and empirical work, nurturing the disruptions in my own understandings and gently pushing me toward exploring new imaginations. That communication needs to be recovered from the large-scale co-optation of communicative spaces and channels is an invaluable learning thread that emerges through my collaborations with each of these dedicated activists. Community organizers on my projects from Gary, Indiana, to Paschim Medinipore, West Bengal, Indranil Mandal, Tony Gillespie, Tracy Robinson, Tafor Bonu, and Delowar Jahan have actively offered visions for academic–community partnerships for the politics of social change. Many community members across the globe, many of them disenfranchised by the very structures discussed throughout this book, have given their labor and knowledge to the making of this book. I am ever so grateful for their work, which is integral to this academic politics of rendering impure the taken-for-granted assumptions of neoliberal organizing.

Mitch Allen at Left Coast Press, Inc. commissioned this series as an opening for new discourses in global health communication. I am grateful to him for believing in the value of this series and in this project as a way for opening up conversations. Thanks also to my series coeditor, Ambar Basu, for the conversations and the collaboration on this project. This book is supported by a grant to CARE from NUS. I am grateful to NUS for the support for this work and for the ongoing empirical projects at CARE.

Family, a space for solace and nurturing, has always been my source of inspiration. I am blessed to have been born in what is described as a joint family in India, with an entire community of uncles, aunts, cousins, nephews, and nieces that give me so much joy. In all of this celebration, my grandmother, Nana, remains a recurring presence. The stories I learned from my grandmother as a child are the sorts of stories that taught me to imagine. Baba's love for books, his activism from the heart, and his participation in communicating for change offered me the earliest lessons in the practical value of theorizing from the heart. Ma steadfastly remains the pillar that guides my moral and intellectual journey, inspiring my curiosity and teaching every day the valuable lessons of care. That my mother believes in me brings the kind of solace that assures the uncertain steps I take into the world. My extended family, Dutta Bari, inspires my imagination. Munna and Susmita offer the joys of laughter and camaraderie, and I am grateful for their unwavering faith in Dada. Vihaan offers inspiration with his ever-expanding vocabulary, his new adventures, and his affection for his jethu. The Banerjees in Gauhati are sources of sustenance, offering a great deal of joy in the everyday celebrations of life.

My wife, Debalina, holds a special place in my journey as a researcher and as a writer. Her steadfast support and love offer the anchor in my scholarly and activist work. That she refuses to uncritically accept the tenets of critical theory offers many a pleasurable Sunday-morning friendly argument, and she pushes me to think harder through my critiques, turning the lens on my own complicity within structures of power. Her everyday presence through the many facets of our lives is the mainspring of my intellectual pursuits. Our son, Shloke, is a wonder who amazes me with his kindness. The questions of my six-year-old, his capacity to love and nurture, and his incredible knack for caring for others are reminders of the beauty of human nature that challenge the basic tenets of the neoliberal model of selfishness and greed. Our daughter, Trisha, came into our life in 2014 as an invitation to new imaginations. Her unfettered smiles that greet me early in the morning, her joyful explorations into this world, and her strong sense of self are intertwined with the stories of change I work through in this book. "What is the kind of world we want to live in?" is a question that Trisha's presence in my life prods me to consider seriously. She inspires me to work with the (im)possibilities of putting theory to work in this complex world of academic–community partnerships.

CHAPTER ONE

NEOLIBERALISM AND HEALTH

Contemporary organizing of health across the globe has been constituted under the framework of globalization, marked by the rapid shrinking of time and space and by the accelerated movement of labor, capital, and resources across global boundaries (Navarro, 2007). Globalization as we know it today has been driven by the political and economic rationality of neoliberal organizing that celebrates individual responsibility, self-care, empowerment, and self-help, accompanied by the minimized role of the state in the delivery of welfare; deregulation of labor, environment, and finance; and stimulation of global commerce and investments through minimization of regulations, tariffs, and subsidies (Brown & Baker, 2012; Dutta, 2008, 2011; Harvey, 2005; Navarro, 2007; Shugart, 2010). *Neoliberalism* refers to a complex web of political and economic thought that considers at its heart the principle of the free market as a driving mechanism for political, economic, and social organizing (Harvey, 2003, 2005), and, therefore, constructs governance in the image of the free market based on an "individualist micro-economic model" (Bourdieu, 1998, p. 9). Under the narrative of the free market, human potential is maximized when the limits imposed by the state are minimized, thus enabling a catalytic climate for growth, productivity, and efficiency.

Although primarily formulated as a form of economic organizing captured in the understanding of a free market as an enabler of freedom, neoliberalism amalgamates political, social, and cultural narratives of organizing within its framework of the free market achieved through the participation of the individual in exchange processes (Brown & Baker, 2012; Moreton, 2009) and through the catalyzing role of the state as an enabler of free enterprise (Harvey, 2003, 2005; Navarro, 2007). The free enterprise of neoliberalism is manifested in the freedom of transnational corporations (TNCs) to trade freely across global borders, serving primarily as a pattern of global organizing that enables the continual accumulation of capital in the hands of the power elite. In this sense then, neoliberalism is a particular form of global organizing backed by powerful global actors with economic resources to shape politics, economics, and social organizing in ways that enable this cycle of continual extraction of resources, accumulation of

Neoliberal Health Organizing by Mohan J. Dutta, pp. 11–50.

capital, and consolidation of power, carried out under the twin narratives of growth and liberty. Communication, working through dynamic processes of assigning meanings, constitutes the framework of legitimacy for global organizing structures, working through public relations, persuasion, and journalism. It is, therefore, vital to interrogate the meanings that circulate in neoliberal formulations of local, national, and global policies. Journalism, public relations, and public communication campaigns are integral to the global diffusion of neoliberal values within mainstream structures. What then are the specific meanings that are given precedence within these mainstream communicative structures?

This book specifically focuses on connecting these meanings that achieve hegemonic status within the mainstream structures of global organizing to questions of health. The hegemony of neoliberalism, I argue, is achieved through *communicative inversions*, the deployment of communication to circulate interpretations that are reversals of the material manifestations. These communicative inversions are fundamental to key disciplinary threads of communication scholarship, constituting communication as advertising, public relations, persuasion, strategic communication, integrated marketing communication, communication management, and communication campaigns directed at changing knowledge, attitude, and behavior through influence. One of the dominant threads of communicative inversion under neoliberalism centers on the organizing role of the state in facilitating the hegemony of the free market. Whereas the neoliberal organizing of the globe is predicated on the communicative circulation of the narrative of minimal state intervention, the materiality of neoliberal organizing is predicated on the powerful imperial role of the United States in protecting internal markets and simultaneously manipulating international financial institutions (IFIs), namely, the World Bank (WB), the International Monetary Fund (IMF), and the World Trade Organization (WTO), to open up markets for U.S. TNCs. Similarly, nation-states across the globe have played instrumental roles in shaping the conceptualization and implementation of the neoliberal model. These communicative inversions are integral to the production of the health inequalities that we witness across the globe. Throughout the book, we will interrogate the discursive articulations, processes, and strategies that are deployed toward reproducing global health inequalities and weakening public health infrastructures.

Yet another element in establishing the power of the global elite in the context of health is *communicative inequality*. *Communicative inequality* refers to the unequal access to sites of discourse, discursive processes, and discursive articulations (Dutta, 2004a). Communicative inequality works hand in hand with material inequality such that the lack of access to material resources mirrors the lack of access to symbolic resources (Dutta,

2008). The voices of subaltern communities are erased from discursive spaces by turning them into subjects of interventions, stripping communities of their agency and of their ability to make meaningful decisions. Techno-deterministic solutions foregrounding innovations and new technologies are directed at subaltern communities, generating new markets for privatized innovations and simultaneously excluding subaltern communities from participatory opportunities. Expert-driven solutions such as building culturally sensitive health promotion campaigns and building cyber-infrastructures and information superhighways offer one-way channels for message dissemination without really creating spaces for listening to subaltern communities or addressing the underlying material inequalities (Viswanath & Kreuter, 2007; Viswanath, 2011). The framing of communicative inequality in the dominant literature constituted within neoliberal logics promotes techno-deterministic solutions without really addressing the underlying material inequalities and without creating spaces for listening to subaltern voices. Communicative inequality thus is constituted amid neoliberal governance as the absence of spaces for voicing community needs, ideas, and imaginations within global discursive spaces. As an exemplar of communicative inversion, these erasures of participatory opportunities for the subaltern sectors are often carried out through technologies of participation that apply tools of participation, collaborative decision making, community engagement, and deliberative democracy precisely to accomplish the preconfigured agendas of the powerful global actors (see the critique offered by Dutta & Basnyat, 2008).

Against this backdrop of communicative inequalities, the health impacts of neoliberalism are witnessed in the weakening of public health programs and resources, the displacement of the poor from their spaces of livelihood, the weakening of local agriculture in the face of large-scale corporate agriculture, the piracy of indigenous knowledge and the corresponding commoditization of health solutions in a global market, the rising inequalities within states, the minimization of economic opportunities for the poor amid structural adjustment programs, growing unemployment, the weakening of unions and organized sites of resistance amid state-sponsored violence, the increasing exposure to workspace risks as the poor subject their labor to exploitation in unregulated spaces, the increasing exposure to pollutants and health risks at global sites of production, and the minimization of opportunities for productive participation at the margins of global economies (Dutta, 2013a, 2013b; Millen & Holtz, 2000; Millen, Irwin & Kim, 2000). Human health is one of the fundamental areas that has been adversely affected by the neoliberal organizing of global politics, economics, and society. What then are the dominant interpretive frames of neoliberalism, and how are these frames connected to health?

Evident in the neoliberal organizing of the globe in the two decades following the introduction of the neoliberal reforms in the 1990s is the dramatic rise in global inequalities. Inequalities are evident both within and across nation-states, with nation-states in Africa experiencing large-scale extraction of resources. The large-scale inequalities evidenced globally are pronounced, with increasing disparities in the distribution of resources between the haves and have-nots (Gershman & Irwin, 2000; Monteiro, Conde & Popkin, 2004; Piketty, 2014). Based on analysis of U.S. income data from 1910 to 2010, Piketty (2014) demonstrates that in the United States, the top decile share in the national income increased from 30 percent to 35 percent in 1970, and to 45 percent to 50 percent in 2010. Moreover, critical to the analysis offered by Piketty is the accumulation of private wealth, measured in the form of real estate, financial assets, professional capital, and net of debt, demonstrating that in Britain, France, and Germany, the rise in private wealth went from one to three times the national income in 1950 to four to six times in 2010. He notes that at the juncture of the financial crisis in the United States in 2008, the upper decile's share exceeded 50 percent of the U.S. national income. Piketty thus offers a twofold explanatory framework: (a) the large gaps in income inequality are tied to the power held by the managerial classes to set their own remuneration, which, in many cases, cannot be correlated with their productivity; and (b) the disproportionate levels of return on capital compared with the growth rate of the economy suggest that inherited wealth has grown at a greater level than economic output has. What then are the systems of global organizing prevailing from 1990 onward underlying the persistently increasing patterns of income and wealth inequalities?

Ample evidence connects income and wealth inequality with inequalities in health outcomes. Moreover, evidence from public health documents the relationship of societal-level inequalities with broader aggregate health outcomes for the entire society. Persistent inequities in health outcomes are observed both within as well as across countries (World Health Organization [WHO], 2008). For instance, infant mortality varies dramatically within countries with the level of mother's education. In Mozambique, babies born to a mother with no education have infant mortality rates greater than 120 per 1,000 live births compared with babies born to a mother with secondary or higher education (60–70 per 1,000 live births). These inequalities are observed in comparison of countries, as well, with infant mortality of just over 20 per 1,000 live births in Columbia compared with the infant mortality of just over 120 per 1,000 in Mozambique. According to the WHO (2008) report, in the United Kingdom the mortality rates among the poorest segment are higher than those in the middle segment, which in turn are higher than those in the least-deprived segment. Marmot (2004) refers to this relationship between social disadvantage and health outcomes as the social gradient in health. Aligned with critical health analyses that point toward broader structures of organizing that constitute inequities in health outcomes, the chapters in this book seek to interpret the structures of organizing that normalize, produce, and circulate inequities in health outcomes. How do these underlying forms of global organizing of resources constitute inequalities in health outcomes? What stories, meanings, and interpretations get circulated within these structures?

In this introductory chapter, I first examine the ways in which global health has been formulated under the organizing principles of neoliberalism and then work through the potential challenges that result from the framing of health as a subject of neoliberal intervention (Dutta, 2008; Youde, 2012). What are the assumptions in the neoliberal organizing of health, and how are these assumptions framed in the health communication solutions? What are the meanings of health that emerge in neoliberal policies and programs, and how are these meanings organized globally? Most importantly, what are the health impacts tied to these policy articulations and the meanings they circulate?

As we read this introductory chapter as a framework for understanding the key principles of neoliberalism, we will first review the literature in critical health communication, identifying the key debates in communication of and communication about health. Our critical reading will examine questions of power and the ways in which these questions of power play out in formulation of policies. Through an emphasis on the meanings that circulate around health, we will attend to the broader structures of organizing within which health is situated. *Structures* refer to the frameworks of organizing material resources that both enable as well as constrain access to these resources. Structures of health constitute resources such as hospitals, education, food, employment, work, and so on, that reflect the ambit of global health inequalities. How then are these inequalities reproduced through the meanings circulated in neoliberal conceptualizations of global health? After taking a close look at the intellectual trajectory of neoliberalism and the key tenets of neoliberalism, we will then examine the role of neoliberal interventions within the broader framework of health. It is my goal to demonstrate throughout this chapter the continuities and divergences between the imperial tropes of development communication in global health and the contemporary epoch of neoliberal health organizing.

Critical Health Communication: Meaning, Culture, and Power

This book is guided by a critical framework of health communication, engaging with questions of meaning, power, and practice of health as understood and disseminated within the structures of globalization (Dutta,

2008; Zoller & Dutta, 2008). Conceptualizing power as structurally situated in relationships, institutions, and networks, critical health communication examines the meanings of health that are circulated globally, and the communicative processes that carry over these meanings in policies, programs, and reports. Attention focuses on discourse and the ways in which language works in health settings to serve the interests of the status quo while simultaneously marginalizing certain sectors of society (Lupton, 1994). Specific interpretations of health are put forth as organizing frames of global governance, framing politics, economics, and society along the lines of these meanings. Examining closely these meanings in relationship to the structural formations that constitute them offers entry points to understanding the processes and networks of control that are intrinsic to the accumulation of wealth and the dispossession of the margins. Aligning this understanding with the context of health focuses attention on the specific forms of communication that are deployed in the privatization of health, normalization of global inequalities, and dissemination of capital accumulating practices that are intrinsically threatening to the health of communities.

In laying the foundations of critical health communication theorizing almost two decades ago amid widespread neoliberal reforms that were taking root globally, Lupton (1994, p. 55) offers the following guiding questions: "In whose interests is the discourse operating? What (and whose) values, beliefs, and concepts are espoused, and what others are neglected? What pre-established knowledge or belief systems are drawn upon to create meaning? What types of social differences are established or perpetuated?" Cultural values, forms of representation, and narratives emerge as the contextually situated sites for the enactment of power, as well as for the consolidation of resources in the hands of the global elite. Practices of health come to be formulated within the narrow terrains of capitalism accumulation and health is turned into a commodity to be exchanged through participation in the market. The depiction of the health consumer as the owner of health accomplishes the privatization of health through a language of participation. Participation in the market is seen as the mechanism for ensuring health. As a consequence, health solutions that are put forth are organized in the logic of accumulation, not as a fundamental human necessity and right. Critical interrogation of the meanings of health attends to the structures of governance through which health is constituted, delivered, and talked about in policies and programs. How health is talked about and the meanings assigned to health are essential to the hegemonic assertion of neoliberal health policies. As Hall (2003, p. 10) notes, "a new neoliberal common sense" has captured the imagination of civil society, having achieved hegemonic status in the everyday organizing and workings of society.

The critical approach sees language and meaning as intrinsic to the policies of health and development that are carried out, and it connects language and meaning to broader social, political, and economic structures. Discourses of health are not neutral, but instead are connected to cartographies of inequality that shape these discourses and are further reproduced through these discourses. Knowledge is central to the reproduction of inequities as it is deployed to consolidate resources in the hands of the global elite. Therefore, critical health communication interrogates the languages and meanings that reside in global discourses of health and the ways in which these meanings are mobilized to reproduce global inequalities. Attention is paid to the structures of knowledge that circulate specific knowledge claims across global networks of power.

In a nutshell, these discourses of health are powerful in perpetuating the dominant taken-for-granted assumptions about structural inequities in distribution of resources. Extending the critical argument within the broader organizing of global political economy, the rest of the book will closely examine the underlying values and taken-for-granted assumptions in health policies, programs, and practices, and the ways in which these values and assumptions reify the structural differentials in local–global distributions of health resources. A key thread that runs through the book depicts the continuity of meanings from the frames of global development articulated in the post–World War II period to frames of meanings that are constituted amid neoliberal narratives of development, depicting neoliberalism as a later manifestation of capitalist accumulation (Amin, 1997; Connell, 2010). Working through these continuities reflects the organizing framework of Western imperial control (primarily the United States in contemporary manifestations) that constitutes the processes of wealth accumulation and unequal distribution of global resources, accomplished through the collaboration between economic, military, and political elites in the global periphery and their collaborators in the metropole (Amin, 1997).

The culture-centered approach emerges out of this critical tradition to suggest that meanings of health are realized at the intersections of structure and culture (Dutta, 2008). Structures, rooted in economic resources, are forms of organizing that enable as well as constrain access to resources. Structures in this sense are material in their nature, interconnected with the resources of everyday living, manifest in access to the various social determinants of health, such as education, income, food, and shelter. Cultures, referring to the shared values, rituals, and practices that connect people within spaces and offer the recipe for action, are realized in their relationship to structures. The shared meanings that circulate within cultures are expressed in relationship to material distribution of resources and, in turn, shape these material distributions of resources. For instance, the dominant ideas of neoliberalism are turned into everyday practices of living through the powerful role of media structures in making familiar neoliberal values rooted in individualism, greed, and selfishness. Agency is enacted as individuals, households, and communities make sense of structures through culturally derived understandings. Meanings therefore are essential to the reification, reproduction, and circulation of specific structural logics, rendered understandable through shared cultural values. Cultural values are continually in flux, shaped by structures as well as integral to the materialization of structures. Agency also offers an entry point into transformative possibilities as new meanings enter into dominant discursive spaces through everyday practices of interpretation as well as through expressively resistive forms of collective action. Agency expresses itself in both working within as well as in working against the dominant structures of global organizing.

In contemporary forms of health organizing that hold a hegemonic position across the globe, the interpretations of the free market, liberty, individual participation, individual responsibility, efficiency, and effectiveness play fundamental roles in the creation and reproduction of health structures. The culture-centered approach suggests that health needs to be understood as broadly being constituted amid the interplays of culture, structure, and agency (Dutta, 2008, 2011, 2013a, 2013b). Therefore, experiences of health are closely intertwined with the organizing of economics and politics: locally, nationally, and globally. Moreover, health is connected with questions of agriculture, food security, displacement, work, education, environment, and opportunities for social mobility. This book will delve into the key terms of neoliberal governance and the ways in which these terms render salient particular frames of health while at the same time backgrounding and/or erasing other ways of interpreting health. That interpretation lies at the heart of global organizing processes will offer a lens for delving into the dominant health communication scholarship to explore the frameworks of health that are salient in this scholarship and the relationship of these frameworks to the normalization of health as an individual resource to be purchased through participation in the market. The goal of the book is to broaden the scope of what we come to understand as health communication, expanding beyond the narrowly conceived individual-based models of health to include questions of agriculture, food security, displacement, work, and environment.

Neoliberalism: Context and Intellectual Trajectory

Neoliberalism underpins contemporary forms of global economic and political organizing under the framework of the free market, connecting global spaces as resources for the investment of global capital and as markets for the global extraction of surplus value by the owners of capital (Campbell and Peterson 2001; Dumenil & Levy, 2005; Rodgers 2001). Dumenil and Levy (2005) outline the propaganda of neoliberalism that utilized the language of the market and private interests to consolidate resources in the hands of the global elite in the form of financialization, simultaneously producing slow growth and unemployment as well as tremendous forms of inequalities across global spaces. Although the rhetoric of neoliberalism portrays a nonintervening state, the state is very much a key factor in neoliberal expansionism, working locally to minimize unions and other threats to capital and simultaneously working globally to expand markets for capital. A key element of neoliberalism is its active role in the promotion of the interests of capital, simultaneously erasing the interests of workers through the weakening of unions and the depletion of state-driven welfare resources. In this sense, neoliberalism as a form of governance works actively to extract wealth in the hands of transnational capital while simultaneously oppressing the working classes, poor, and subaltern sectors, weakening the organizing capacity of these classes through state repression.

Neoliberalism achieved its hegemonic status first in a top-down U.S.-backed experiment in Chile that was orchestrated by the collusion between the Chilean elite and U.S.-backed diplomatic and military interventions (Dutta-Bergman, 2005; Harvey, 2003, 2005), followed by large-scale economic reforms introduced in the United States and UK in the 1980s in response to the oil-crisis-induced "stagflation" (Gourevitch, 1984; Prasad, 2006). It was later consolidated in the form of the Washington Consensus in the 1990s, subsequently disseminated across the globe through the powerful roles of the IFIs, namely, the World Bank (WB), International Monetary Fund (IMF), and the World Trade Organization (WTO) (Dutta, 2011; Peet, 2003). The global power of neoliberalism as an organizing concept has been structured within the powerful roles of academia and think tanks in shaping economic policy making in the form of the influences of Thomas Freidman and the Chicago School, think tanks such as the American Enterprise Institute and the Institute for Economic Affairs, governments in the global North (primarily the United States and the UK), IFIs, and a rising class of elites across the globe (Harvey, 2006). Global economic policies have been shaped by the structures imposed by the IFIs, which in turn have been influenced largely by the governments located in the global North, primarily the United States, working hand in hand with local elites across nation-states (Harvey, 2006; Yergin & Stanislaw, 1999). Neoliberalism therefore, is also a project of imperialism, facilitating the transfer of vast amounts of resources from the poorer sectors of the global South to elite local actors and to the United States (Saad-Filho & Johnston, 2005).

Initially working through development promotion initiatives that were directed toward promoting the rationality of the free market conceptualized within the ambits of capitalism and democracy through development aid funded by the United States Agency for International Development (USAID), the global diffusion of the free market agenda was accelerated through the 1990s through the structural adjustment programs (SAPs) imposed by the IFIs as a condition for loans under the neoliberal regime. The post–World War II period experienced the ascendance of U.S. hegemony through the promotion of violence often coded in the rhetoric of democracy promotion, accompanied by the role of the USAID in actively promoting the opening up of nation-states to U.S. financial capital, liberalizing international credit and financial markets (Panitch & Gindin, 2005). U.S. banks investing in foreign governments exerted the power of U.S. hegemony in demanding rates of return that were higher than the domestic rates within the United States, pushing the countries thus toward default. Simultaneously, the risks of investment were effectively shifted to the countries taking the loans from the financial institutions who were making the loans, thus pushing the countries of the global South toward debt traps (Harvey, 2006).

Against this backdrop, the advent of neoliberalism was marked by the emergence of the nexus between the United States, IFIs, and international banks in actively pushing the agenda of opening up markets as the condition for debt resettlement for nation-states that had defaulted (Harvey, 2006). As demonstrated in the case of Mexico in its debt rescheduling bid after the economic crisis of 1982–4, nation-states receiving loans from the IMF were required to implement structural reforms in the form of privatization, relaxed labor laws, and cuts in welfare expenditures by the state (Gowan, 1999; Panitch & Gindin, 2004, 2005). The IMF emerged as a key player in the global political-economic landscape in pushing the agenda of neoliberal reforms across the globe. As Harvey (2006) observes, the IFIs formulated and imposed neoliberal reforms such as the surrender of local assets to foreign companies at "fire-sale prices" (p. 24) as the cost of repayment, irrespective of the effect of the interventions on the health and well-being of local populations. The hegemony of neoliberalism was achieved through the powerful role of transnational capitalism in shaping the U.S. and UK agendas, in shaping the agendas of the IFIs, and in working collaboratively with local elites across the globe who benefited tremendously from the inequitable distribution of power in political and economic spheres. In instances where the neoliberal experiment was resisted by people experiencing the effects of inequalities, the local–global elite networks actively worked through violence, repression, and persuasion to thwart such resistance (Dutta, 2013a, 2013b).

The power of neoliberal hegemony to shape global social and economic policies left key imprints on human health. Governance structures and structures of delivery of health were and continue to be fundamentally reconfigured under neoliberalism through expert-driven technologically mediated solutions offered through the framework of the market, conceived in the form of technological innovations, and implemented through the participation of the individualized subject in the exchange of health resources. Simultaneously, state-driven programs of welfare and delivery of health resources are depleted. Public health programs and structural health capacities to meet the basic needs of the poor are undermined as resources are invested into privatizing of health as a commodity. The large-scale inequalities produced by neoliberal interventions are closely related with adverse health outcomes for poorer communities and poorer health at aggregate levels for communities with high levels of inequalities.

Knowledge Networks and Meaning Frameworks

Neoliberalism, as a framework of political and economic organizing, works on the basis of configuring solutions in the hands of experts, privileging technologies as solutions, and connecting social, political, and economic organizing to notions of the free market (Plehwe, 2013). Essential then to the meaning structure of neoliberalism is the active role played by expert knowledge networks in actively positioning the free market as the solution to global political, economic, and social organizing. This expert-driven framework of knowledge production lies at the heart of neoliberal interventions and is well captured in the early roots of neoliberal expansionism in the active role played by think tanks and academic networks of intellectuals, seeking to recover the liberal Western tradition as a general principle of governance in opposition to the state-planned models of socialism, collectivism, planning, and Keynesianism (Cockett, 1995; Mirowski & Plehwe, 2009; Plehwe, 2008, 2013). The Mont Pèlerin Society, a network of elite academics in philosophy, history, sociology, and economics, accompanied by businessmen, politicians, and journalists, articulated the foundation of neoliberal thought, coming together as an intellectual collective to push the fundamental concepts of individual freedom and liberty in economic organizing (Plehwe, Walpen & Neunhöffer, 2007). These concepts were presented through knowledge networks as constituting a desirable frame for reorganizing the global order, connecting ideals of individual life to broader principles of economic organizing.

The neoliberal thought collective was formed in interpenetrating networks between academe and think tanks, supported by collectives of businesses and foundations (Cockett, 1995). Think tanks such as the

Institute of Economic Affairs (IEA), the Center for Policy Studies, and the Adam Smith Institute played foundational roles in shaping the policy advocacy functions of the neoliberal collective and in carrying out the agendas of the collective in shaping key opinion leaders and public opinion. Philanthropy played a key role in shaping the neoliberal thought collective, with business conservatives pouring money into the neoliberal networks to shape the guiding assumptions of economic policies and programs. Banks and financial sectors played powerful roles in the shaping of neoliberal ideas and in pushing the formulation of specific meanings of the free market that would then form the basis of neoliberal propaganda. Knowledge in this sense was actively constructed.

Political leaders looked to the think tanks for research and guidance in pushing free market reforms. In the UK, Member of Parliament (MP) Geoffrey Howe, who became an avid reader of IEA publications, corresponded with Arthur Seldon, editorial director of IEA, to gather data to shape his free market advocacy and critique of universal welfare services (Cockett, 1995, p. 170). Consider, for instance, the following memo written by Joan Culverwell, the secretary of IEA director Ralph Harris, to Harris and Seldon:

> Geoffrey Howe rang up re: the Crossman pension Scheme. There are many people in the City who are now aware of what is happening. Geoffrey is writing a pamphlet with Norman Lamont about the pension Scheme, and he thinks it may not be too late to start front and popular movement against it.
>
> A.S. [Arthur Seldon] Have you any information, articles, publications etc. you could send him which would help to throw this pamphlet together? When the time comes he want to tell H.M. Opposition to vote against it and why. He would like the information *urgently* please.
>
> R.H. [Ralph Harris] Geoffrey suggests that perhaps half a dozen of you (us) could start up some organization (i.e. like Wincott, I.U. [Independent University of Buckingham] etc.) into which you could get your teeth and call it something like STOP- Save the Occupational Pension. He would like to discuss this seriously with you . . . would you ring him please. (Cockett, 1956, p. 170)

The production of knowledge thus was intrinsically tied to the shaping of the political process and political outcomes. Research produced through IEA was explicitly directed at shaping public policy in the image of the free market. The advocacy and public relations functions of knowledge production are critical to note, with pamphleteering serving as a key mode for shaping public attitudes and values and for influencing existing belief structures.

As depicted in the conversation thread, establishing the hegemony of neoliberalism was critical to the production of knowledge directed at explicitly challenging social welfare services and state provision of resources for public health and well-being. The ideological ascendance of neoliberalism continued this thread of market-driven reform, centering the discourse of the market to delegitimize public health services, health care resources, and public welfare programs, depleting state resources for health programs, and constructing health in the language of the market. Simultaneously, neoliberal reforms were formulated under the principle of organizing growth through the use of credit, the powerful role of the technocracy, and the weakening of unions that were seen as threats to the functioning of the market (Fourcade-Gourinchas & Babb, 2002; Loriaux, 1997).

The advocacy function is often played by experts working at the free market think tanks such as the Heritage Foundation and the American Enterprise Institute (AEI) in the United States and IEA in the UK, systematically producing knowledge with the intent of establishing neoliberal hegemony, disseminating ideas grounded in free market principles of individual responsibility and ownership (Carroll & Carson, 2006). Consider, for instance, the following lessons on welfare reform offered by Robert Doar (2014) from AEI in the *National Review*, citing the example of his work with the New York City welfare system:

> *Always promote personal responsibility.* The minute an applicant believes that government will solve all of her problems, she loses. Accepting responsibility for one's own future is the vital first step to moving up . . . This is especially true when it comes to getting a job. Lots of "programs" want to say that they got a participant a job, or "placed" a certain number of people into employment. But for entry-level jobs, the person who gets the job is the person who gets the job, and the sooner the clients and the caseworkers realize that, the better.

The meaning that is central to the politics of welfare reform is grounded in the articulation of individual responsibility as a solution to poverty. This emphasis on individual responsibility as a solution to poverty is then circulated in policy and public circles with the goal of impacting the ways in which policies are talked about and the ways in which these policies are implemented.

Other elements of welfare reform pushed forth by the AEI include encouraging married two-parent families, developing greater mechanisms of surveillance and monitoring, and promoting every kind of economic development idea that promised job creation. Erased from the discursive space are the structurally situated exploitations of the working poor who struggle to make ends meet and simultaneously don't qualify for welfare resources because of eligibility criteria, the lack of minimum-wage policies that ensure basic economic access among the working poor, and the absence of organizing spaces among the working poor to demand for greater access to economic resources. Instead, the organizing of the poor is weakened in order to create resources of cheap labor for the owners of capital. Consider further the following articulation by AEI expert Doar in response to the minimum-wage policies being supported in New York City in 2014:

> Will the city's economy continue to outpace the rest of the country's? Given the new mayor's support for policies such as mandated paid sick leave and a higher minimum wage—both of which make workers more expensive for businesses to employ—I am doubtful that job growth will remain as strong as it has been. As a result of these changes, the number of people classified as poor may grow in New York City. This may come as a surprise to some, given Mayor de Blasio's progressive rhetoric. But it shouldn't be surprising at all—there is a long history of progressive policies' losing ground in the war on poverty.

Essential to the idea of poverty in neoliberal thought is the weakening of the organizing capacity of the poor and the bargaining capacity of the poor to secure greater resources for the work they do. Minimum wage and sick pay leave are portrayed in the free market ideology as being antithetical to the interests of the poor. Paradoxically, therefore, poverty emerges into the discursive space as a narrative for pushing policies directed at securing cheap and unorganized labor for the owners of capital. Poverty ironically serves as an organizing trope for the bolstering of neoliberal policies and programs that lie at the heart of producing poverty.

The Role of the State

The crux of the neoliberal narrative hinges on the minimalist role attributed to the state, based on the argument that the market will take care of human, societal, cultural, political, and economic needs (Peck & Tickell, 2002; Ward & England, 2007). Yet the dominance of neoliberal hegemony lies essentially in the powerful role of the state in simultaneously rolling back public welfare resources, weakening the organizing capacity of labor, minimizing regulations of corporates, and, for states in the powerful global North, in increasing the networks of the state in pushing for opening up global markets for TNCs located in the global North (Dumenil & Levy, 2005). For Peck and Tickell (2002), neoliberalism is the "rolling back" and "rolling out" of state formations, reorganizing the state to serve the interests of the owners of capital. The state has played an active role in aligning itself along the lines of capitalist interests, working actively to redraw spaces, forms of organizing, and institutional arrangements to deliver policies and programs serving the interests of capital (Peck, 2001; Peck & Tickell, 2002).

As an integral player in the redrawing of policies to align them to serve the interests of capitalist hegemony, the state reconceptualizes the interpretations of the public and private to move resources into the private sector, and to increasingly consolidate power in the hands of transnational capital (Colas, 2005; Peck & Tickell, 2002). For Ward and England, neoliberalization is a "process of state restructuring" (2007, p. 15). Rather than playing a minimalist role, the state actively participates in serving and protecting class interests, simultaneously restructuring itself and its deliverables to secure, create, and disseminate new markets for the owners of capital. The powerful role of the state is evident in the role played by USAID in prying open global markets for U.S.-based TNCs, albeit under the aegis of promoting free trade under an ideology of growth. Development interventions carried abroad have been justified as instruments for promoting global free trade, whereas in practice these interventions have been instrumental to the development of markets abroad for TNCs located within the state. The creation of open markets for U.S.-based TNCs in the global South have been framed as altruism that would promote development while in essence the opening up of markets in the global South have resulted in the weakening of local industries, the weakening of the public sector, the removal of regulatory policies protecting health and the environment, the weakening of labor laws and capacities to unionize, the rise in unemployment, the weakening of wages, and the weakening of collective bargaining and organizing capacities.

The integral role of the state to the functioning of the market perhaps became most evident during the financial crisis that began in 2008. Starting with the initial phase of the financial crisis to its current manifestations across global spaces, the state emerged as a key player orchestrating the bailouts of banks and leveraging resources to bail out these banks. In one of the greatest ironies of neoliberalism, taxpayer money has been directed by state actors toward saving big banks without much public accountability. In other words, the dominant actors of the free market economy that have advocated for tax cuts and minimum state intervention have benefited the most from state interventions targeted at protecting the big banks from failure. These state interventions therefore have been essential to the framework of the contemporary manifestations of neoliberalism, on one hand precisely using the state to serve the interests of capital and, on the other hand, pointing to state bureaucracy, red tapism, and inefficiency as convenient discourses to push for minimum state regulation and accountability for the large corporate structures.

At times of trouble, as reflected in the recent financial crisis, when public opinion rises against the tremendous consolidation of resources in the hands of the power elite and against the fundamental injustices of neoliberal policies as depicted in the recent bailouts in the United States, the state emerges as a specter of violence. State-owned police and military are deployed to protect and perpetuate the interests of transnational capital. As witnessed with the recent protests on Wall Street, resistance to the commoditization of public spaces and resources is thwarted through the deployment of state power. Violence as an instrument of neoliberalism keeps intact the punctured discourses of neoliberalism and continues to perpetuate these prevailing logics of neoliberalism in spite of growing evidence that point toward the failure of neoliberal rhetoric of growth, efficiency, trickle-down economics, and progress.

The Politics of the Market

The global hegemony of neoliberalism is closely intertwined with the local hegemonic assertion of neoliberal governance through the ascendance of the market. The assertion of neoliberalism as a form of rule is tied to the power interests of large owners of capital and corporate managers, linking the politics of neoliberalism to the interests of capital (Connell, 2010). The market becomes the conduit for the delivery of basic capacities of health. For instance, conversations about questions of health care access privilege the notion of the market as the organizer of health care access. Universal access itself becomes a mechanism for ensuring consumers of health, mediatized through mechanisms of the market.

The framing of human beings as consumers privileges the market-driven logic of health. For instance, the Affordable Care Act (ACA) introduced in the United States within a broader imperative of securing universal access to basic health care resources was reshaped into a narrative of the market, emphasizing the individual patient as a consumer of health resources driven toward making optimal health decisions in the marketplace. For example, the health insurance marketplace within the ACA frames health care access as a question of choice, offering a portal for health care consumers for comparing various health insurance schemes.

> The Health Insurance Marketplace is designed to make buying health coverage easier and more affordable. The Marketplace allows individuals to compare health plans, get answers to questions, find out if they are eligible for tax credits for private insurance or health programs like the Children's Health Insurance Program (CHIP), and enroll in a health plan that meets their needs. (www.hhs.gov/healthcare/insurance/index.html)

The framing of the possibility of universal health care within the United States in the ambits of the insurance marketplace depicts the powerful role of the politics of the market, constructing health as a commodity in the market connected with consumer choice rather than as a universal human right.

This thread of commoditization of health becomes evident in the mainstream literature in health communication through the ascendance of social marketing as an organizing framework for developing persuasive health communication strategies. Understanding health as a commodity can be critical to the deployment of traditional marketing strategies to produce and circulate persuasive health messages. Referring to a condom promotion campaign using the social marketing strategy in Madagascar, Evans, Longfield, Skekhar, Rabemanatosa, Reerink, and Snider (2012, pp. 330–331) note:

> The purpose of brands and branding is to organize and frame choices—to buy a product, to use a service, or to live a physically active lifestyle or use condoms. Brands use symbols and imagery—colors, shapes, sounds—to organize our potential choices and frame the benefits of a particular product, service, or behavior has to offer. Nike has the "swoosh" and Coca-Cola has the distinctive red color and shape of its iconic bottle. In recent years, public health social marketers have begun to use similar approaches, as in campaigns such as *truth* and *VERB* in the United States.

The formulation of health is tied to the analogy between health behaviors and products or services. Health is understood as an individual choice presented within a marketplace. The adoption of that choice then is tied to the persuasive impact of messaging, symbols, and images, placing active lifestyle and condom use amid brands such as Nike and Coca-Cola. The Nike "swoosh" and the distinctive red color of Coca Cola are offered as symbolic inspirations of effective social marketing strategy rooted in meaningful branding.

Deregulation and Weakening of Labor

The processes of deregulation that lie at the heart of neoliberal restructuring emphasize the creation of enabling environments for the generation of profits (Brenner et al., 2000). The free functioning of the market is accomplished through the deregulation of labor laws such that TNCs can operate in conditions that enable the maximization of profits. The rush toward minimal labor regulation is constituted within a competitive environment where economies compete with each other to invite transnational capital. As a result, many nation-states across the globe establish strict controls on labor organizing in order to attract foreign investments, and simultaneously deregulate labor, with minimal legal protections for workers. Long working hours are symptomatic of manufacturing units in the global production chain, accompanied by low wages for the many workers housed within these units.

Neoliberal reforms implemented in the United States and UK, for instance, were accompanied by strong anti-labor programs that sought to minimize the threats to productivity posed by labor. The removal of unions and collective bargaining rights are intrinsic to the creation of a climate of optimal production. Neoliberal organizing processes introduced across the globe directly target labor unions with the goal of minimizing their bargaining rights if not completely eliminating them. National labor unions co-opted as an extension of the state render silent the dissenting voices of workers.

The weakening of labor organizing and the deregulation of labor have direct implications on health by impacting wages, working hours, working conditions, occupational health and safety, and broader environmental conditions within which workers and their families live. For instance, in the *Maquiladoras* set up on the U.S.–Mexico border, the dumping of wastes into the Rio Grande tributaries has contributed to the contamination of the Rio Grande with hazardous wastes, with high levels of toxic organic discharge, as well as metals such as chromium, nickel, and lead (Lewis, Kaltofen & Ormsby, 1991).

Liberty, Trade Liberalization, and Health

The essence of the principle of liberty is private property (Cockett, 1995). The ability of the individual to hold private property and to trade it in the global market is seen as the embodiment of liberty. The liberalization of global trade processes is enforced and policed by the WTO, formulated as a global structure for ensuring the smooth flow of goods and services. The WTO emerged from the General Agreement on Trade and Tariff (GATT) that was signed by twenty-three countries in 1947, driven by the free trade ideology that if every country specializes in goods that it can produce efficiently, exchanging these goods with other countries in a free market, the cost of production will be globally reduced and every nation-state participating in free trade will economically benefit.

The free trade principles reflected in the WTO are also integral to the various free trade agreements between nation-states. Instruments such as the North American Free Trade Agreement (NAFTA) are critical to the minimization of barriers to trade between regions. When trade barriers are sought to be minimized through these agreements, some of the key sites of intervention are regulatory policies related to health, agriculture, food, labor, and environment, privileging the business needs for productivity. The language of liberty applied in the context of global neoliberal interventions connects the logic of the market to the broader notions of human existence and global political structures.

The Neoliberal Organizing of Health

The earliest frameworks of health communication under capitalist market promotion emerged in the form of population control programs that were directed toward the Third World, often tying the logic of economic growth to development and situating population control as essential to economic growth (Dutta, 2008; Speidel, Sinding, Gillespie, Maguire, & Neuse, 2009). Development was framed in the narrow terms of economic growth, and population growth was seen as a barrier to development. The health of individuals and families in the Third World was tied to the logics of economic growth, suggesting that population control would foster greater health through household economic prosperity as well as nation-level economic growth. Health, juxtaposed amid population growth, was narrowly conceived within the framework of population control.

These population control programs, a large number of which formed the foundations for the development of the earliest communication knowledge, formulated in the form of state-based aid given out by the United States (USAID) and UK (Development Foundation [Dfid]), were directed at the Third World as state-based mechanisms for promoting liberty and freedom in the newly emerging economies, tied to the logic of promoting economic growth and a capitalist framework of development. In other words, development, economic growth, and population control emerged as markers for pushing the liberal democratic framework across the global South, accomplished through the imperial networks of the United States and UK, often embodied in development interventions supported by the USAID and DfiD. The population control programs often worked simultaneously as tools for prying open markets in the global South (Dutta, 2008).

The movement from the development framework to the neoliberal framework of global health witnessed increasing emphasis on privatization as a mechanism for delivering health. As the capital-driven fundamentalism of development promotion gradually turned to the principles of free market, the logic of capital-driven health was reorganized into narratives of the free market, technological interventionism, individualism, efficiency, expertise, and security. These meanings of market-driven health and individualism were both consistent with earlier notions of growth-driven development and simultaneously divergent from the earlier development paradigm.

Health in the Free Market

An excellent example of the neoliberal framework of market-driven health care is evident in the discourses around privatization of health care in the United Kingdom in the 1960s. IEA, created by capitalist interests in Britain in 1955 as the advocate of neoliberal reorganizing of political economy, was playing a key role through its manufacturing of theory and research pieces as well as through public-opinion-shaping pieces written by IEA member journalists. In addition, politicians who were members of IEA were playing formative roles in the dissemination of free market thought in policy circles and in shaping policies accordingly. Consider the following letter written by IEA member and politician-cum-businessman Sir Keith Joseph in the UK to Arthur Seldon (cited in Cockett, 1995, p. 168):

> Any shift in health from public to private or partly private finance is going to be greeted with allegations that we are robbing the large predominantly less well-off public clientele of irreplaceable doctor and medical man hours in favour of private and generally better-off clientele. The essence of the case as I see it is of course that in fact private demand at market rate will draw back into practice extra doctors who are now giving up either medicine or this country. But that would take a little time to prove and the first year of any such scheme would be bound in fact to reduce the amount of medical attention available to the public. I want to put into your head *the political difficulty of the short term and say* how helpful it would be if in some way we could establish that in fact more doctors would be available both to public and to private practice if we opened up health to a limited extent to the market.

Evident in the letter is the advocacy function of the politician working with the research produced by IEA. The role of research is defined in the context of a political advocacy function seeking to redefine health within the logics of the market. Here, market fundamentalism expresses itself in the assumption that opening up health care to the mechanisms of the market would drive more doctors into the health care system. The goal of research then is framed in terms of advocacy, shaped by the need to prove or demonstrate how opening up health to market processes would make more doctors available to both private and public practice.

Communication has emerged as a key player in the neoliberal organizing of health in the language of the market. For example, the U.S. health industry including large pharmaceuticals, insurance firms, and hospitals paid over $380 million campaigning against the ACA introduced by the U.S. president Barack Obama. The campaigning money went into the lobbying industry, with the deployment of approximately six lobbyists for each member of Congress to oppose and/or modify various elements of the policy (Crouch, 2011). Campaigning primarily meant investments into the reelection funds of sitting members of Congress, thus practically investing private sector resources to purchase political decisions along the lines of private interests. As a result of the intense lobbying by the health industry, the ACA shifted dramatically from an initial national health insurance fund to a mandatory private health insurance policy, thus essentially creating new customer bases for the insurance industry.

Health as Technological Intervention

The narrative of development exerted the hegemony of the global North/West (United States/UK) through development programs that were invested in the diffusion of technologies of progress such as birth control and agricultural innovations. Across these threads of development, health was conceived of as an outcome of technological interventions, expressed in health outcomes attached to population control and its later version of family planning. The emphasis therefore of global relationships was constituted within the context of sources and recipients of technological interventions, with health being narrowly framed within the structures of technologically deterministic solutions (Murphy & Gryboski, 2005). Knowledge, attached to the scientific and biomedical discourses of technological innovation, was situated and produced in the global North, directed as development toward the global South with or without collaborations with local elite actors as co-participants in the diffusion of innovations.

Attitudes, as reflections of predispositions toward these technologies of modernity conceived within the development framework, are seen as targets of interventions. Changing existing attitudes of traditional societies is seen as being instrumental to the process of development. In his dissertation titled "Mass Media Participation and Modernization: A Causal Analysis," directed under the guidance of Professor Wilbur Schramm, U.S. professor Robert Hornik exemplifies this worldview. In a section titled "What Is the Process of Change?" Hornik (1973, pp. 21–23) observes:

> The traditional man perceived a slowly changing world. Relatively unsophisticated information processing skills are sufficient. There is no constant need to transform the rules by which the world is understood. In time, whether through city visits with friends who have had those exposures, he perceives that there is information that his worldview did not include, and still later he perceives that there is information that is inconsistent with his worldview. These inconsistencies need to be resolved . . . As the traditional man repeatedly enters into the cycle two results occur. First he is more willing to risk exposing himself to information, information that may be inconsistent with his worldview . . . Secondly he gains practice in processing information dynamically. He is able to accept larger and larger inconsistencies and resolve them, changing his processing rules. In terms of the definition presented above, he is becoming modern.

Becoming modern is reflected in a communication process that is captured in the resolution of incongruities, catalyzed by exposure to the technologies of modern mass media. Among the various barriers to the direct correspondence between exposure and modern information processing are intelligence, commitment, and the limited nature of mass media in continuing to provide inconsistent information. Worth noting are the racist depictions of traditional societies as primitive, rife with primitive states of information processing and cognitive capacities that are central to the narrative of development. Communication as a marker of forms of information processing delineates the modern subject from the primitive/traditional subject targeted through technological innovations.

Neoliberal health interventions in the global landscape continue to reify this primitivizing logic in creating global markets for technologies of health, positioning these technologies as solutions to poor health (Suggs & Ratzan, 2012). For example, technologies of family planning, repositioned from earlier top-down forms of population control, are reframed within neoliberal frameworks of social marketing that emphasize interpersonal communication, confidentiality and privacy, informed choice, individualized care, dynamic interaction, avoiding information overload, and using and providing memory aids (Murphy & Gryboski, 2005). Communication is framed as the delivery of information on the technologies of health, such as information on effectiveness, side effects, advantages and disadvantages, how to use, when to return and what to do about complications, and prevention of sexually transmitted infections (STIs).

Similarly, neoliberal interventions emphasizing individual choice in adoption of technologies frame communication as information dissemination, social marketing, data-driven market segmentation, program management, audience targeting, consumer-driven targeting, and so on, all constituted in the realm of disseminating technologies of health (such as condoms, oral pills, injectables, and intrauterine devices) (Fikree, 2005). Although the language of individualized choice and empowerment inundate the neoliberal framing of health technologies, the top-down development thinking of technology diffusion continues to form the cornerstone of global public health communication, creating new markets for the technologies of health that are presented as narrow solutions to health.

> Communication is a key process underlying changes in knowledge, attitude, and health behavior (preventive and curative). The channels for the communication can occur at all levels—personal, family, community, the health sector, and mass media. Furthermore, this communication can be spontaneous at the personal, family, and community level, or be planned as part of an information, education, or behavior change communication strategy implemented by government or nongovernmental organizations. The expected outcome of these spontaneous or deliberate information strategies is improved knowledge, attitude, and behavior so as to eliminate misperceptions or inappropriate knowledge regarding reproductive health and reproductive health services. (Fikree, 2005)

The reframing of population control as family planning continued to embody the top-down technologically deterministic solutions of reproductive technologies, with individual choice taking center stage, simultaneously outlining the role of communication in changing existing misperceptions and/or inappropriate knowledge. Local knowledge is seen as a barrier to the adoption of the prescribed technology, and communication is framed as a technology that diffuses the innovation through appropriate mapping of audience needs, contextual complexity, and community needs.

For neoliberal governmentality, the formulation of technology as a solution to health individualizes the locus of decision making, approaching health inequalities as products of differentials in access to information and communication infrastructures (Suggs & Ratzan, 2012). For instance, noting the correlation between health inequalities and communication inequalities, Viswanath (2011) suggests the need for investing in cyberinfrastructure through public–private partnerships with an eye toward addressing inequalities:

> Investment in infrastructure deployment is expensive, and the potential of future return on capital is one critical consideration that the private sector takes into account. Public–private partnerships that brought utilities such as electricity and water to rural areas in the U.S.

> could serve as one exemplar model to make the deployment of cyber-infrastructure economically viable. (p. S247)

Technology as a solution to health becomes evident in the digital divide projects funded by the National Cancer Institute (NCI) in the 2000s (Kreps, 2005). For instance, the NCI Cancer Information Services (CIS) initiatives, such as the CIS New York State, bring together public–private partnerships to make basic cancer information accessible in community computer centers in Harlem, New York. The techno-deterministic solutions toward health inequalities erase the broader structural features of environments, social organization, and economic institutions that shape inaccess to health resources. They also downplay the structural features of environments that play instrumental roles in shaping health outcomes. Erased are questions of inequalities, inaccess, unemployment, weakening of labor, and so on, that are produced by technologically driven neoliberal reorganizing of spaces. What are the conditions of labor through which the technologies are produced, and what are the health impacts of these conditions of labor? Also erased are questions regarding the health impacts of the technologies that are disseminated in underserved communities as elixir to communicative inequalities.

Instead, the individualization of health solutions in the realm of building cyberinfrastructure capacity places the technology in the driver's seat. Ironically and similar to other forms of neoliberal interventions that propose to tackle the very inequalities of health that are produced by neoliberalism, addressing health inequalities becomes tied to investments in technologies rather than addressing the underlying deep-seated structural features of the environment. The inequitable structures of access and disparities in access to fundamental structural resources are erased from the discursive space, also simultaneously erasing discussions of inequalities that are produced by technologically driven organizing. Within these dominant imaginations of neoliberal interventionism, technologies become platforms for promoting individualized health behaviors and lifestyles rather than emerging as spaces for interrogating the power structures that constitute health inequalities. Instead, public–private partnerships embodying the neoliberal restructuring of health are proposed as solutions for building the technology infrastructure. Ironically, it is worth noting that these public–private partnerships lie at the center of the privatization of health across the globe, therefore being at the heart of global inequalities in health outcomes.

Health as an Individual Artifact

In global narratives of health running from the development narratives immersed in Cold War imaginations to contemporary neoliberal forms of health interventions, health resides in the individual. This primary interpretation of health as an individual artifact therefore privileges method, design, intervention, and evaluation that is directed toward the individual and his/her ownership of health. In health communication, the dominant paradigm of health communication campaigns is directed at knowledge, attitudes, and behavior of the individual, based on the assumption that encouraging individual level preventive behaviors would lead to better health outcomes. In the face of the consistently large health inequalities experienced across global spaces, health communication interventions seeking to address these disparities primarily focus on the level of the individual. As a result, the dominant structures of organizing and systemic structural patterns of inaccess to social determinants of health remain erased from discourses, policies, and programs.

The conceptualization of health as an individual resource and responsibility is further evident in the concept of individual competence in the global model of health communication and competence put forth and widely used by the Johns Hopkins Bloomberg School of Public Health, drawing from extensive reviews of existing health communication theories and integrating lessons learned. Individual competence is defined in terms of intrinsic interest in health issues and valuing of good health, openness to communicating about good health in familial settings, and the degree of self-confidence in one's own ability to achieve health outcomes. Health competence is seen as playing an important role in the context of individual health competence outcomes such as health information seeking, change in or reinforcement of health beliefs and attitudes, health information recall, health literacy, perceptions of social support, reduced stigma attitudes, and increased self-efficacy. Further, these health competence outcomes are likely to lead to health behavior change.

In the global model of health communication and competence, individual competence is theorized in relationship to community competence, service competence, political competence, and global competence. Community competence taps into the participation in community improvement efforts by members of the community, community-wide social norms around health behaviors, and a collective belief in the community's ability to tackle health challenges. The community is theorized as a product of individual members, and community participation is understood in relation to individual outcomes. Community competence conceptualized in terms of social capital then is likely to result in engaged communities. Communication ranging from interpersonal communication to mass media communication and interactive communication are seen as playing important roles, and communication strategies such as social marketing, entertainment-education, web-based marketing, and social media are deployed to catalyze community competence. Although the emphasis is shifted to the level of the community, worth noting here is the emphasis on the individual as the participant in social networks and in community-driven processes. Tools of social marketing and entertainment-education are seen as catalysts of community participation, with the community working as an important rung in the individual behavior change process, conceived under the broader logics developed and articulated by campaign planners. The nature of the intervention remains constrained to individual behaviors, simultaneously erasing discussions of the broader structures that organize health inequities.

Similarly, the concept of service competence referring to improved interpersonal communication and counseling, client-centered outreach, and correct use of technical skills taps into the individual communication skills of the provider. Political competence reflects the political interest and commitment in addressing health challenges, tapping into the climate for the development and implementation of appropriate health policies and the adequate investment of resources to enable implementation of policies. Global competence taps into the international relationships among nation-states and between public and private sectors to foster positive health outcomes. Although the framework works through multiple levels of competence, the emphasis is ultimately on individual behavior change. Health is owned by the individual, and it is through his/her participation that better health is secured. This same logic of individual behavior change dominates much of the paradigm of health communication campaigns. Lessons from social marketing turn the individual consumer into a decision-making agent who needs to be persuaded into adopting the proposed behavior change. The framing of the targeted individual as the consumer further consolidates the marketization of health, where individual behavior is a commodity with attached values and costs. The goal of persuasion then becomes one of framing the value of the proposed behavior through branding, pricing, placement, and product promotion strategies.

The Logic of Efficiency

The delivery of health is conceptualized within a narrow framework of efficiency, thus creating room for a business model for defining, implementing, and evaluating health. In setting up the stage for privatization, networks of knowledge in the form of think tanks, consulting firms, and paid academics are recruited by transnational capitalists to construct narratives of state inefficiency. The documentation of bureaucracies and inefficiencies in state-based processes create openings for importing logics of privatization into health and other basic resources of living such as food, water, energy, and air. Worth noting, however, in this rhetoric of efficiency is the absence of evidence that critically evaluates the claims of efficiency that are made by the narratives of privatization. Is private management of basic resources such as food, health, energy, water, and air indeed efficient in its delivery of these resources? Moreover, the premise of greater access created by privatization is often countered by the evidence base that documents decreasing opportunities for access once pivotal basic resources have been privatized. The foregrounding of questions of efficiency work hand in hand with the erasure of questions of fundamental access, basic rights to public resources, and the inequalities in the distribution of these basic resources. Should efficiency be the primary framework through which fundamental resources are evaluated? What other frameworks are available for debate and consideration? Interrogating the taken-for-granted notions of efficiency opens up possibilities for creating alternative systems of health organizing grounded in notions of universal access, collective ownership, and shared collaborations.

The Technocratic Elite

The continuity between the development framework and the neoliberal framework of global organizing of health is manifest in the hegemonic role of experts as the developers, designers, implementers, and evaluators of development policies and programs. Neoliberalism catalyzed the dominance of an elite coterie of global and local experts who are in charge of setting the development agenda as well as implementing and evaluating specific programs reflecting this agenda. The emphasis on technology as the solution to health problems is framed within the historic articulation of development as achieved through the diffusion of technologies as innovations. The framing of health solutions as innovations creates ready-made markets for health experts who thrive economically on the basis of the distinction between the modern and the primitive.

An entire coterie of managerial classes is invented through the logic of development rooted in neoliberalism. For instance, the large organizational structures of funding agencies such as the USAID, Ford Foundation, and DfiD; the structures of university research and implementation departments such as the JHU/CCP; and the structures of global and local NGOs working on health implementation projects are sustained by the depictions of felt needs in underserved communities. The deployment of professional experts as the ones creating the solutions also devalues the participatory decision-making capacities of communities, moving most of the resources allocated in health projects into the hands of outside and local elite actors. Technologies of neoliberalism create conditions for experts at far-off locations to design, implement and evaluate local projects based on little contacts with communities, while local community staff are paid to organize communities, set up community meetings, and create community-placed channels for the dissemination of the innovations conceived by the global experts. Interrogating the assumed power of experts creates opportunities for interpreting alternative frameworks of knowledge creation grounded in local community voices, community access to knowledge, and community participation in processes of everyday decision making that impact community health.

Health and Security

Global health serves as an umbrella term for neoliberal interventionism that frames health in the language of security and turns it into a site of profiteering (Everts, 2013; Gostin, 2009; Sparke, 2009). Terms such as *emerging infectious diseases* and *global pandemic* are deployed to suggest the temporal and spatial nature of new health threats that are connected to globalization, placing these threats under the surveillance and management networks of global structures such as the UN and WHO. Critical interrogations of global interventions on emerging infectious diseases interrogate the portrayal of severity attached to the health threats as compared with the actual magnitude and severity of the health issue (Caduff, 2010). Depictions of severity attached to the health threats circulate extreme responses of public anxiety, and serve as the foundations of health organizing directed at effective global management so as to promote the security of boundaries, simultaneously offering the impetus for logics of privatization by creating new markets of surveillance and new markets for the global pharmaceutical industry (Caduff, 2010; Gallaher, 2009; Michaelis, Doerr & Cinatl, 2009). The securitization of health has resulted in the deployment of material resources under the structures of the military-industrial complex, shifting economic resources for health into the realm of the military and surveillance industries (Sastry & Dutta, 2012).

Moreover, the framing of health as a security threat to the flow of transnational capital has worked as a trope for justifying aggressive interventions that are directed at leaving intact the structures of elite control, simultaneously locating power in the hands of transnational elite to dictate global health agendas. The consolidation of power in the hands of the military further reifies the role of the state as an instrument of control, often deploying security as a trope to justify the transformation in organizing of resources. The shift in the meaning of health as a human right to a security threat justifies a variety of forms of exercise of power, targeted at managing the threat at an individual level.

The management of security threats is tied to articulations of spaces as modern and primitive, where trajectories of movement resulting from the very economic structures of neoliberalism are sought to be managed through border control, development of measures of security, and development of appropriate strategies for control. The geography of disease vectors is expressed in the location of the disease within national boundaries, once isolated in East Asia, again isolated in Africa, deploying the material structure of disease control to contain the disease (see, for instance, Chitnis, 2012). The management of security threats in a neoliberal narrative deploys the racist tropes of imperialism that mark the other as a site to be controlled.

Neoliberal Interventions and Health

Across the globe, the advent of neoliberal interventions has contributed to large-scale inequalities, resulting in consistent gaps between the rich and the poor. Polarization of economies has resulted in the increasing disenfranchisement of the poorer sectors of the globe, with the global movement of vulnerabilities across national boundaries, even as a significant proportion of people in China and India have moved from the income of less than $1 per day into the $1 to $2 per day category, ameliorating somewhat the trends in global inequalities because of their large numbers. Neoliberal interventions have been associated with the increasing disenfranchisement of the poor in terms of the lack of absolute access to resources and the growth in inequality within nation-states, as well as the growth in inequality between nation-states.

Food Insecurity

One of the key elements of health that emerges in narratives of the poor in the backdrop of global neoliberal interventions is the lack of access to adequate, safe, and healthy food, situated amid the rapid privatization of food resources, the privatization of land, and the wholesale technologization of agriculture. Food has been turned into a global commodity to be transacted and exchanged through the global marketplace. The state, especially the powerful states of the global North, has played a pivotal role in pushing the privatization of agriculture. A predominant form of U.S. interventionism guiding the development logic sponsored by the USAID was the diffusion of agricultural technologies in the form of genetically modified crops. This diffusion of agricultural technologies through state-driven development interventions worked hand in hand with the project of capitalist expansion, seeking to reorganize spaces into global markets, incorporating universities such as Cornell University and research centers such as the Bangladesh Agricultural Research Institute into public–private partnerships.

Since the early history of communication research, communication played a central role in the formulation of development interventions, with communication technologies working to disseminate agricultural innovations designed in the global North into markets in the global South. The technological solutions to agriculture created commodity markets for agriculture, also simultaneously working through agricultural technologies to turn agriculture into a commercial sector. The commoditization of food resources therefore was integral to the imperial logics of development. Inherent in this development logic was the notion of bringing about development through the dissemination of agricultural technologies that were thought to pave the way for the green revolution. The cultures of recipient societies located in the global South were constructed as traditional and as devoid of agency. Therefore, communication technologies were conceived as instruments for modernization, bringing about shifts in values and attitudes, fostering openness to innovations, and eventually facilitating the large-scale adoption of innovations, simultaneously fostering forms of dependence on both agricultural as well as communication technologies. Agricultural technologies (such as the hybrid seed) and communication technologies (such as the radio or television) serve as tools of modernity. The shift from the development model of agricultural innovations to the neoliberal model of innovations was witnessed in the large-scale commercialization of the agricultural sector at a rapid pace, the turning of agricultural technologies as instruments of private profit, the large-scale adoption of public universities and research centers as spaces for researching, evaluating and diffusing privately owned technological innovations, and the continued use of development agendas to push these privatized agricultural technologies. This shift, however, was also a continuation of an imperial logic manifested in early global development interventions.

As a consequence, for many agriculturally-based economies in the global South, the formulation of the neoliberal agenda resulted in the switch from food-based agriculture, where farmers spent their resources growing food, to cash-based agriculture, where the goal of agriculture was transformed into the production of raw materials in the cash economies of the global market. Locally sustainable forms of agriculture were being replaced with top-down technological innovations, with limited impact studies on health, environment, politics, economics, and local sociocultural fabrics. The marketization of agriculture therefore incorporated it into the global market economy, connecting it to profits, technologies of neoliberal growth, and fluctuations in the global market. The large-scale adoption of technologies called for large investments into the irrigation systems, seed systems, and fertilizer systems. Farmers, especially small-scale farmers in the global South, depend on debts taken out from local moneylenders in order to fund the agricultural innovations, simultaneously turning them as vulnerable to global economic fluxes, fluxes in commodity prices and demands, and flows of financial capital. Debts taken out to invest in corresponding technologies such as large-scale irrigation systems, pesticides, and so on, place the farmers further in cycles of poverty. Moreover, with the absence of locally-based knowledge on the growing patterns of the agricultural technologies, shifts in local weather patterns may correspond with failures in crop cycles, leaving farmers even further trapped in cycles of poverty. The large-scale suicide of farmers in India in communities that were targeted as sites of adoption of Monsanto-produced/owned Bt technologies (primarily Bt cotton) points to the violence embodied in the large-scale corporatization of agriculture and the accompanying processes of turning agriculture into a commercially driven economy.

Yet another aspect of neoliberalization of agriculture is evident in the deployment of corporatized knowledge to systematically steal local forms of knowledge rooted in communities in the global South, turning such knowledge into commodities to be exploited by pharmaceutical transnationals, protected by the trade-related intellectual property rights (TRIPS). As a policy framework, TRIPS works primarily through the erasure of local claims to knowledge production, and turning these claims into private commodities that can be transacted by TNCs in global markets.

The SAPs imposed by neoliberal interventions have been accompanied by forced reduction of tariffs on imported food supplies, leaving local farmers vulnerable to global agro industries that produce, market, and distribute food on the mass scale. Simultaneously, state-based subsidies for farmers in the global South have been forcefully minimized to further push the opening up of markets even as powerful nation-states in the global North have continued to maintain strong subsidy programs and tariffs to protect farmers in the global North. The implementation of neoliberalism as a form of governance therefore has been uneven and unequal, with contradictory logics being deployed simultaneously to push the agendas of powerful interests mostly situated in the global North. Farmers left vulnerable to these uneven flows of agricultural produce, resources, and policies have been forced to migrate to urban centers in search of jobs, producing urban vulnerabilities and exploitable sources of labor.

Displacement

The dispossession-based model of neoliberal interventionism works through the transfer of resources from the poor and the underserved sectors into the hands of the owners of capital, justified in the naturalized meanings of the market and in the accumulation of surplus (Dutta, 2008, 2011; Harvey, 2006). The state in this case works hand in hand with IFIs and transnational capital in ensuring the dispossession of the poorer sectors and in the transference of resources from the poor to the rich. The narrative of development framed within articulations of economic growth is deployed to consolidate land in the hands of the power elite. Harvey (2006) maps out the trajectory of development by displacement, noting the corresponding processes of accumulation and devaluation by dispossession. The large-scale industrialization, financialization, urbanization, and technologization of the globe at a rapid pace, constituted amid time space compression, have resulted in the rapid displacement of rural and indigenous communities from their spaces of livelihood, displacing them from their homes, resources of food, and cultural resources, justified by the need for national economic development and conceptualized in discourses of economic growth. In the state of Gujarat in India, paraded as the marker of vibrant growth-driven development branded through glossy events management programs carried out by the global public relations giant APCO, large-scale displacements of agricultural communities have been carried out in order to secure land for the owners of capital. What is powerful about this displacement-based development is the seduction of the growth-driven narrative that erases the materialities of displacement, loss, and violence experienced by the displaced communities.

The exploitation of natural resources to be fed into economic growth has been intertwined with the corresponding displacement of rural and indigenous communities living in these spaces, normalized as integral to the logics of surplus accumulation. These large-scale displacements of the poor reflect the uneven patterns of development that constitute the neoliberal narrative, formulated in arguments of economic growth, progress, and poverty alleviation, while simultaneously extracting resources from the poor into the hands of the elite sectors. This neoliberal articulation of growth as development naturalized through dispossession is an accelerated manifestation of logics of imperialism that interpreted the colonization of spaces as essential to capital accumulation. Observes Harvey (2006, pp. 91–92):

> Natural resources and other conditions in nature provide for the possibility of rapid surplus production so that open access to and control over resource rich sites becomes a shadow form of accumulation through appropriation. The perpetual search for natural resources of high quality that can be pillaged for surplus and surplus value production has therefore been a key aspect of the historical geography of capitalism.

The large-scale and rapid appropriation of natural resources has been integral to neoliberal globalization, as projects of natural resource exploration and energy creation have been integral to the cataclysmic character of surplus accumulation. Across spaces in the global North, such as in the case of the laying of the Keystone XL pipeline that would carry tar sands from Canada to the United States, to spaces in the global South, such as in the case of the Niyamgiri Hills in Odisha (Dutta, 2013a), the exploitation of natural resources, the conversion of these resources into usable commodities, and the delivery of these resources and commodities to sites of consumption have resulted in the large-scale displacement of communities, along with the production of adverse health effects in these communities.

The displacements of the poor from their spaces of livelihood have been complemented by the migration of the poor as cheap labor to sites of mining, industrialized agriculture, industrialization, and so on, often exposing the poor to greater health risks. The working conditions in the mines are threatening to health. Similarly, the working conditions in industrialized agricultural sites are exploitative, with extremely low wages for long hours of work done on the field. Exposure to fertilizers and insecticides add other health risks to the nature of work being done.

Health is shaped within these displacements as communities living in poverty struggle to generate sources of income and sustenance in the newly configured spaces. The experiences of health and development amid displacements are antithetical to the rhetoric of development crafted within neoliberal interventions and within the promises of development by displacement. For instance, in describing the Bauxite mining project and the accompanying distillery carried out in the Niyamgiri Hills of Odisha, India that threatened to displace communities of Dongria Kondh, an indigenous community residing on the Hills, Vedanta Aluminum, a British mining transnational, appeals to the narrative of development and poverty alleviation.

> Vedanta recognises that the socio-economic situation of the Dongria Kondh is characterised by poverty and lack of access to sustainable livelihoods that is beyond what is usual, even in this poor region. They have major development needs and while they have a distinct way of life and cosmology relating to their lives in the forest, they are becoming more acculturated and want a better life. (Vedanta, 2010, p. 26)

The framing of the Dongria Kondh as a community living in poverty serves as the backdrop for introducing the development needs of the community and the want for a better life, which in turn serves as justification for the mining and distillery operations. The rapid pace in exhumation of natural resources, the suspension of community processes of decision making, and the simultaneous deployment of force are integral to the neoliberal project, framed paradoxically as the necessary resource for sustainable livelihoods.

The erstwhile narrative of development that inundated post–World War II discourse is rearticulated within neoliberal imaginations of development, delivered through the privatization of resources, the delivery of employment, and the development of infrastructures such as roads and bridges that are intrinsic to the implementation of the project. The story of development draws on the imagination of the nation-state, understanding development in a narrow sense of exploitation of natural resources, accumulation of surplus, and generation of wealth. The rhetoric of development in the Niyamgiri Hills is marked by its departure from the lived experiences of health, dispossession, and disenfranchisement among the communities living in the local spaces of Niyamgiri. The framing of land grabbing within the story of development is reflected in the following statement made by Juergen Voegele, director of the Agricultural and Rural Development Department at the World Bank:

> When done right, larger-scale farming can provide opportunities for poor countries with large agricultural sectors and ample endowments of land. To make the most of these opportunities, however, countries will need to better secure local land rights and improve land governance. Adopting an open and proactive approach to dealing with investors is also needed to ensure that investment contributes to broader development objectives. (Transnational Institute [TNI], 2013, p. 5)

Securing investors to land is seen as intrinsic to achieving the development objectives. As noted by the TNI report, arguments of scarcity are put forth as justifications for land grab and accompanying displacements, undermining the questions of resource distribution that essentially underlie food insecurity. Worth noting here is the displacement of meaning, where the meaning of development is framed under the language of investment, capitalization, and financialization, and broader questions of development in terms of access to basic resources are simultaneously erased.

That most forms of large-scale land acquisition benefit the rich farmers and those with resources while simultaneously marginalizing smallholder farmers and landless farmers whose lands are acquired remains erased from the discursive space. Also erased are broader questions of health and well-being with the resulting disenfranchisement of the poorest of the poor in rural communities. The form of development that gets articulated within the narrative of land grab therefore is a form of capital accumulation that catalyzes growth through the dispossession of the subaltern sectors. The framing of agriculture as a source of investment constitutes agriculture as a private enterprise, positioned as a solution to global food insecurity in spite of the evidence that ironically suggests that turning agriculture into a capitalist enterprise is the very cause of food insecurity. Finally, the depiction of poor countries with vast endowments of land rhetorically paints a picture of vast amounts of empty and investable land being available for investment in the poorer countries in spite of the reality that much of the land in the global South is occupied by farming communities that live, work, and grow food on this land.

In Uganda, similarly, large areas of land have been acquired for the production of cash crops as a mechanism for attracting foreign investment, allowing foreign companies to move into land areas for large-scale palm oil plantations, carbon offset treat plantations, and oil drilling (National Association of Professional Environmentalists, 2012). A study of the effects of land acquisition on health in the Kalangala palm oil project in the Bugala Island in Lake Victoria funded by the WB and the International Fund for Agricultural Development (IFAD) documents adverse health effects such as breathing difficulties, skin problems, and headaches, as well as the increased risks of HIV/AIDS with the movement of migrant workers into the region.

Risks

The large-scale movements of people from rural and agrarian spaces into global spaces of production for the neoliberal economy have both created new spaces of risks and simultaneously removed these risks from discursive spaces. Through uses of various forms of control, bodies are managed at global sites of production where cheap labor is increasingly extracted through production cycles to create increasingly productive and efficient processes of extraction. Risks are circulated in production processes of geosecurity and geostrategy, turning the interpenetrating sites of bodies and risks as targets of profiteering. Risks embody the structures of biocapitalism, forming the sites for the development of new biotechnologies, technologies of surveillance, and technologies of crisis response. In communication, entire sectors of communication technologies are constituted around the management of crises and response to crises.

Violence

As noted earlier in this introduction, the threat of violence lies intrinsic to the processes of consolidation of power in the hands of the transnational elite (Giroux, 2006). Police, paramilitary, and military forces are continually deployed by the state apparatus to thwart voices of resistance. Popular protests against the large-scale inequalities produced by the neoliberal reforms are silenced through the deployment of violence (Dutta, 2013b). The enactment of violence is legitimated not only through the machineries of the state but also through the privatization of control in the form of private security forces deployed by the state. Private security firms and mercenaries are recruited by the state and paid through public resources in order to carry out violence. State resources are invested into TNCs transacting in these technologies of violence. Correspondingly, once the violence has been carried out, state resources are deployed toward rebuilding, implemented in the form of large infrastructure projects and opportunities for investments.

Violence is not only enacted within internal spaces of policing in nation-states but is also an instrument for creating global crises in the form of imperial invasions, building markets, securing resources such as oil, and opening up opportunities for investments. Imperial wars such as Operation Iraqi Freedom and the invasion of Afghanistan are carried out in the name of democracy promotion. As in the early democracy promotion efforts in Chile, Nicaragua, and the Philippines, current imperial invasions of nation-states in the global South are tied to the agendas of creating markets in these spaces. The very processes of creating war are themselves revenue-generating mechanisms, creating large markets for transactions in weapons. Moreover, once spaces have been brought under control, constitutional reforms are leveraged as strategies for transforming the political economy of invaded spaces. After the invasion of Iraq, the United States leveraged the crisis scenario in Iraq to carry out large-scale neoliberal reforms of the political economy (Harvey, 2005). The narratives of terror and security are deployed simultaneously to normalize violence.

Similarly, strategic opportunities such as the popular resistance against authoritarian forms of governance abroad are leveraged as mechanisms for disseminating the neoliberal ideology. Nongovernmental organizations (NGOs) such as the National Endowment for Democracy (NED) are allocated resources to destabilize governments in the name of democracy promotion, funding global–local networks of NGOs and creating elite bases of support for neoliberal ideas. Funding is channeled into nation-states in the global South in order to foster pro-market reforms, married with arms supplies and militarization. As demonstrated in the case of Libya, local struggles become opportunities for exploitation in the hands of global power structures, legitimating the use of violence to secure spaces for neoliberal reforms globally.

Work

As noted in the earlier section on deregulation of labor laws, the vulnerable conditions of workers in the special economic zones (SEZs) is evident in the poor working conditions in the Maquiladoras on the U.S.–Mexico border, where labor laws and environmental protection laws are both weakened by neoliberal interventions facilitated by NAFTA. SEZs emerge in neoliberal spaces of production as opportunities for maximizing productivity, efficiency, and profits, often reproducing poor working conditions for workers who work extreme hours on tedious jobs with very little pay. Labor therefore is seen as a resource that can be exploited to the utmost capacity to maximize production processes and to streamline these processes with an eye toward efficiency. As will be demonstrated in Chapter Seven, even in the contexts of technology-driven work in unregulated global spaces, workers experience high health risks, including stressors from long hours on repetitious jobs, stressors from job vulnerability, musculoskeletal problems from repeated movements, and so on. Neoliberal instruments such as trade agreements and treaties are deployed in order to create effective and profitable spaces of production at the cost of the health of workers and labor rights.

Poor working conditions emerge as central to lived experiences of workers working on global construction jobs as urban infrastructures expand. Worker deaths from falls and workplace accidents speak to the high risks embodied in work. The large-scale displacements of people in the global South brought about by the structural adjustment programs fostered migrations to spaces of work at urban sites of production, fostering vulnerabilities of health tied to work. Displaced communities of women and men work in a variety of high-risk jobs, including work as sex workers, in the mining industry, in the construction industry, and in the many SEZs of manufacturing. Collective organizing capacities, collective bargaining and labor laws are seen as barriers to processes of production.

Education

Education as a fundamental resource is a social determinant of health, correlated with an array of health outcomes. Lower educational levels are correlated with poorer health outcomes across a variety of contexts. The global hegemony of neoliberalism is played out in the large-scale privatization of education across global spaces, turning education into a commodity for corporate profits. Rather than build public infrastructures for basic education, the networks of development institutions, global foundations, and states have increasingly pushed for the deployment of private delivery models. For instance, the Gates Foundation spearheaded extensive reforms in education in the United States, directed at privatizing education and turning education into a market commodity. Experiments with privatized models of education seek to frame education as a choice, and the citizen becomes a consuming subject who must enact her or his choices. Education, increasingly framed as a commodity, has emerged as a site of profiteering, simultaneously being limited to those who can afford the structures. Moreover, the privatization of education has been accompanied by accumulating student debts constituted in the backdrop of massive unemployment among educated youth and the absence of opportunities for securing economic access to resources.

Lack of Access to Health Care

One of the key areas of neoliberal transformation overseen by the WB is the reorganization of global health care. Starting in the 1990s, the WB sought to restructure health care systems globally, with an emphasis on privatizing health care. It introduced the ideology of neoliberalism into health care through its 1993 World Development report, titled "Investing in Health." The report constructed health as a private resource and health care as a private good (Waitzkin, 2011). The WB report pointed to inefficiencies in the organization of health care and suggested market reforms, competition, incentives for private insurance, and privatization of health care. Shaped by powerful transnational interests in the health sector, particularly the managed care lobby, the WB introduced logics of efficiency as the primary interpretive frame to justify the privatization of health care, simultaneously downplaying state-based public health infrastructures as inefficient. Managed care TNCs generated large revenues, such as the Sul America Seguros Corporation of Brazil, half-owned by the U.S. TNC Aetna, which generated single-year revenues of more than $1.2 billion in Brazil. These WB-introduced health reforms made health care inaccessible to lower-income populations across global spaces and simultaneously weakened public health infrastructures. The increased administrative and management costs of the privatized managed care organizations shifted resources away from clinical services. WB-introduced reforms reconfigured health care in the privatized logic of the market.

Conclusion

Unfortunately, much of the scholarship within the mainstream literature that we come to identify as health communication is situated within neoliberal imaginaries that privilege the individual as the locus of decision making. When I consider my own ideological training within this enterprise of theorizing predicated upon the individual as the locus of decision making, the powerful role of interpretation in shaping knowledge claims becomes evident (see Dutta, 2004b). In my early work, across a number of studies on health information seeking reporting analyses of the national-level LifeStyles data gathered in the United States (Dutta, 2004b), I observed systematic patterns of differences in health information seeking. Individuals more interested in health, categorized as health-oriented individuals, were also more likely to seek out health information and participate in health-promoting behaviors (Dutta, 2004b). The interpretation I offered to this observation focused on the individual, interpreting the observations in terms of individual differences and failing to connect these observations of individual differences with broader structural patterns of organizing of health. The analysis I offered thus failed to situate the empirical observation to broader structures within which health, meaning, information seeking, and attitudes are organized. Now part of the problem of theorizing in this sense is its theoretical mapping that inherits the psychologized framework of communication seeking to render transparent individual beliefs, attitudes, and behaviors as targets of communication interventions.

The other part of the problem arises from the individualized methodology of survey and experimental research in this tradition that treats the individual as the unit of analysis. The hegemony of individualism is intrinsic to the theorizing, measurement, and application of health communication campaigns that consider as the unit of analysis the individual and targets his or her lifestyle and health behaviors as sites of interventions. Critical and cultural interrogations of health, biomedicine, and health communication ought to offer entry points for closely understanding the ways in which communication is intertwined with the knowledge claims we make and the material health implications of these knowledge claims. Responsibility is individualized, narrowly constructed within the selfish and individualistic logics of self-care, disconnected from relationships, communities, and broader networks of collective belonging. The understanding of responsibility in the realm of the individual is mediatized through consumption and participation in the free market, simultaneously marked by irresponsibility in commitments toward others, particularly the disenfranchised. The ethic of caring for future generations, taking responsibility for the health of broader global communities, and taking responsibility for the health of the earth are subsumed by the self-care narrative.

This book will offer a framework for closely looking at the meanings, interpretations, and discourses that are circulated in establishing the hegemony of neoliberal thought. The power of neoliberal organizing depicts the twin processes of consolidation of power in the hands of the transnational elite and the simultaneous localization of neoliberal interventions within the ambits of culturally specific reforms. Meanings therefore serve as powerful sites for mobilization of specific sets of ideas that serve the agendas of transnational power. Chapter Two interrogates the framework of development, attending to the ways in which the narrative of development has operated at the center of neoliberal organizing, offering the rationale for neoliberal restructuring of global organizing processes. Chapter Three looks at the powerful role of foundations as key players in the global health arena, followed by Chapter Four, which looks at the interplays between the state and the private sector. Chapter Five attends to the roles of civil society and dominant logics of democracy as instruments of neoliberal reordering of global relationships. Chapter Six explores the symbolic and material articulations of security that constitute global relationships and networks of governance. Chapter Seven examines the roles of military and communication technologies deployed toward servicing the organizing logics of neoliberal hegemony.

CHAPTER TWO

DEVELOPMENT COMMUNICATION INTERVENTIONS AND IMPERIALISM

The earliest ideas of development were founded on the imagination of the "other" that needed to be developed through interventions carried out by benevolent development interventionists. This other was most often defined as the traditional subject constituted in opposition to the developed citizen of the West, marked by the lack or absence of development as conceptualized through the lens of policymakers in the United States and UK. Race configured implicitly into the earliest notions of development, as epitomized in the seminal work of Max Weber (1905) on the Protestant ethic, suggesting that development and innovation were intrinsic to Protestantism and to accompanying notions of progress, as opposed to primitive communities elsewhere that were hardwired to be stagnant and static, thus serving as sites of anti-progress that needed to be transformed. Implicit in the ideas of Weber was the depiction of the colored societies of the Third World as primitive and in deficit of the essence of innovation and progress of the white societies of the United States and UK. These societies elsewhere were considered traditional or backward because they lacked the ethic and character needed for development. Inherent in the work of Weber was the fundamental understanding of modernization as a trait, equated with rationality, and imbued with characteristics of hard work, goal-driven pursuit, efficiency, and rational accumulation.

The economist Walter W. Rostow (1960) of Yale suggested the "stage model" of development, noting that economic development took place in five stages, moving from "traditional society" to "development." Conditions for "takeoff" needed to exist in traditional societies for them to embark on a path toward modernization. Then came the actual "takeoff," followed by "drive toward maturity," and finally "development." In this linear movement from traditional society to development, development could be measured by the gross national product (GNP) of a nation-state. Similar ideas connecting the structures of underdevelopment to inherent individual, societal, and cultural traits were formulated under a dominant ideology of development. Modernization was established as a universal marker for societal progress, achieved through the adoption of technology. The development industry therefore was founded on this ideology, intrinsically tied to the

Neoliberal Health Organizing by Mohan J. Dutta, pp. 51–90.

portrayals of an "unmet need" that could then be fulfilled by the industry through its knowledge of science, technology, and social scientific principles of persuasion, together constituting the axes of modernization.

Communication emerged on the foundations of these core principles of development. The disciplinary foundations of communication were laid out in the conceptualization of directed social change that would bring about development (Dutta, 2011; Dutta & DeSouza, 2008; Melkote & Steeves, 2001). Persuasion emerged as the overarching frame for converting target audiences of development interventions into adopters of development technologies. Culture came to be theorized in the narrative of development as a reflection of backwardness, depicting the traits of traditional societies that needed to be transformed through directed communication interventions disseminating the technologies of modernization. Culture was theorized in this dominant narrative of development as a stable characteristic of a geographically bound population, reflected in its shared values, rituals, and practices, and in need of the new technologies of modernization. These values, rituals, and practices were conceptualized as static characteristics of the culture and therefore were established as the targets for development interventions because they were barriers to the adoption of technology. In this sense then, culture was synonymous with the undesirable characteristics of a target audience in an undeveloped community that stood in the way of development. The development paradigm functioned through an impetus to change economic productivity, limit population size, and diffuse technologically mediated solutions to agriculture.

Health was one of the intrinsic markers of development, with some of the earliest development communication campaigns having been configured under the framework of population control. Development communication campaigns were also health communication campaigns, with the health of populations being conceptualized as intrinsic to the development logic (Dutta & DeSouza, 2008). Budgets directed for health-based development efforts are primarily framed within the ambit of population control. Based on the notion that controlling population growth would bring about economic development in the Third World, development interventions planned by U.S. and UK development agencies and targeted at the Third World focused on disseminating contraceptive technologies and health information among the poor masses. These population control interventions carried the Cold War logic of early U.S. communication research, extending the logic of promoting U.S. geosecurity and capitalist framework abroad through the promotion of family planning. Promoting family planning was conceived as a strategy for controlling the large reproducing masses in the global South that posed as threats to U.S. geosecurity. Moreover, the emphasis on large family sizes as impediments to development defined in terms of economic growth shifted attention away from questions of resource distribution and economic justice.

Another area that emerges as a core area of development communication drawing on the logic of promoting global health is agriculture (Shiva et al., 1991). Investing in agricultural technologies is seen as the route to development, with an emphasis on addressing global problems of hunger. With an expert-driven model that privileges agricultural technologies, development interventions sought to diffuse agricultural technologies in the global South (Rogers, 1983). Inherent in the diffusion of innovations framework that guided the agricultural technologies was the assumption regarding the inherent advantages of these technologies. The Cold War logic continued to be reiterated in the agricultural innovation programs based on the assumption that disseminating agricultural technologies would bring about economic growth and address geosecurity concerns of the United States.

In this chapter, I will argue that the advent of neoliberal governance in this sense is a continuation of the Orientalist Cold War ideology, emerging as a framework for managing global health through a coterie of experts and technocrats that are created with the goal of developing top-down expert strategies for population control and pushing technologically driven agricultural solutions in the global South. In this sense, the development narrative is a key thread in neoliberal governance, continuing the ongoing agendas of population control and agricultural innovation diffusion, albeit reconfigured under the purview of the private sector and public–private partnerships. The global spread of neoliberalism as a universal organizing framework for political and economic governance is spearheaded by development agencies such as USAID, and international financial-economic organizations such as IMF, WTO, and WB.

Development, Health, and Economic Growth: A Linear Narrative

Communication scholarship and practice in the formative years originated from the Cold War agenda into the development agenda, framing the problem of communication as one of bringing about planned social change in the Third World (see Shah, 2011). Cold War sensibilities dominated the development narrative as development was seen as a strategy for countering the communist influence in the newly liberated nations of the Third World, achieved through the twin agendas of population control and agricultural development. In his depiction of the Cold War ideology in the modernization paradigm, Shah (2011) notes in *The Production of Modernization*, that a package of Western governance, industrial organization, values, and general lifestyle were offered as the irresistible pathway to development. The work of social scientists was intrinsic to the prevailing Cold War ideology of development, producing knowledge directed at disseminating innovations in population control and agricultural development.

Therefore, the goals and framework of social change were constituted within the dictates of changing peasant societies of the Third World through top-down interventions from the West. Everett Rogers, one of the earliest proponents of this paradigm, wrote about the importance of modifying peasant attitudes and behaviors, constituted within the Cold War rationality of minimizing the threat to U.S. geosecurity. The rapid growth in large numbers of populations in the newly decolonizing nation-states in the global South was seen as a threat to U.S. geosecurity, with the large populations seen as the recipe for recruiting these Third World masses into communist and revolutionary movements in the global South (Hartmann, 1995a, 1995b). The social sciences, and more specifically the communication sciences, were specifically situated within this agenda of understanding communicative processes within the ambits of human behavior, influence, and persuasion directed at top-down population control (Dutta, 2006). Population control then was clearly established as a mechanism for maintaining U.S. hegemony and its framework of global capitalist control through the containment of population growth threats (Dutta, 2006, 2008; Horn, 2013). The funding for population control under the aegis of USAID, the Rockefeller Foundation, and the Ford Foundation played key roles in achieving the global hegemony of the market-driven model of political-economic organizing, with health serving as the anchor.

The continuity of the linear narrative of development from the earliest days of communication and development/health communication work to the neoliberal forms of global governance is well captured in the slogan "Modernizing the Middle East," which resonates through the subtitle of Daniel Lerner's book *The Passing of Traditional Society* (1958) and the headline of a December 2002 news story on CBSNews.com outlining the Bush administration's plans for Iraq and the broader Middle East (Shah, 2011). The depiction of the Third World as the site of development, with a large "unmet need," becomes the basis for neoliberal interventions carried out through social marketing and entertainment-education programs, funded through private–public partnerships, corporate social responsibility programs, and development-directed efforts of market promotion and privatization in the health sector. The overarching framework of diffusion of innovations offered the conceptual structure for mapping out the pathway for the diffusion of the innovation, conceptualized in the centers of modernity and directed toward audiences in the undeveloped and underdeveloped geographic spaces (Rogers, 1962, 1983, 1995).

Population control has occupied the heart of the narrative of development and health communication, serving as the basis for the development of practice and theorizing in the effects tradition of health communication. This linkage is well captured in Everett Rogers' foreword to the book *Health Communication: Lessons from Family Planning and Reproductive Health* (Piotrow et al., 1997), referring to the powerful national family programs carried out by Population Communication Services under the aegis of Phyllis Tilson Piotrow and colleagues:

> *Health Communication* centers on the lessons learned about effective family planning communication over the past 15 years, during which Population Communication Services (PCS) has been involved with national family planning programs in some 50 developing nations. PCS is a program in the Center for Communication Programs for the Johns Hopkins University's School of Hygiene and Public Health. Staffed by over 100 professionals, PCS works closely with governments, nongovernmental organizations, and commercial firms in developing countries to help design, implement, and evaluate family planning communication programs . . . I recommend *Health Communication* to scholars, students, and program officials who want to know how human fertility behavior can be changed through strategic communication. Here, writ large, is the inside story of how adequate funding over a sustained period, applied by a dedicated staff of able people using strategies based on research, is helping to solve one of the world's gravest problems. (pp. xiii–xv)

Health takes the place of population control. Communicating about health is about controlling population growth, with population control communication and health communication being interchangeable. In this section, I will argue that the Cold War narrative of population control continued to emerge in neoliberal interventions of health spearheaded by the mix of development organizations, international foundations, private corporations, nongovernmental organizations, and local governments. The role of development agencies such as USAID continued to be central to disseminating and implementing the agenda of population control albeit reconfigured in the language of empowerment, choice, and family planning (Dutta, 2006, 2008; Horn, 2013).

Another powerful site of development interventions is constituted in the domain of diffusing agricultural technologies in the form of innovations in seeds, irrigation mechanisms, fertilizers, pesticides, and farm machinery. Fundamental to the diffusion of agricultural innovations was the linear narrative of progress set up on binaries of primitive and modern. For health communicators, the narrative of the "green revolution" is a key site of interrogation because of the public relations discourses of positive health effects of access to food circulated by an entire industry of development communicators juxtaposed against the backdrop of the experiences of food insecurity, impoverishment of the rural poor, and food crises associated with large-scale dissemination of technology-driven agriculture, which, in turn, influence health in most basic ways.

Close interrogation of the "green revolution" narrative circulated as a transformative story of the way in which technology triumphed over nature by changing India from the world's "begging bowl to a bread basket" (Agarwal, 1979, cited in Holt-Gimenez & Patel, 2009, p. 32), suggests that the extensive and rapid diffusion of agricultural technologies produced dramatic health effects ranging from health inequalities, weakened community ties, and community strife to Sikh-on-Sikh violence, problems of alcoholism and drug dependency, and farmer suicides (Association for Democratic Rights [AFDR], 2000; Gill & Singh, 2006; Shiva et al., 2002). The propaganda of uncharted agricultural growth, food production, poverty reduction, and hunger alleviation is reworked under neoliberalism to call for a new media "Green Revolution 2.0," reworked as an instrument of expansion of corporatized agriculture into new spaces in the global South, such as Africa (Cullather, 2010).

Population Control: Controlling the Dark Masses

One of the earliest forms of imperial control carried out through development communication interventions took the form of population control. Inherent in the idea of population control was the emphasis placed on controlling the reproduction of the colored races as an instrument for promoting geosecurity and economic growth. Drawing on the Malthusian (1798) idea of the *Bell Curve*, the earliest ideas of population control were based on "eugenics," encouraging more children from the fit and fewer or no children from the unfit, thus engineering the evolutionary development of the human species (Mosher, 2008). Margaret Sanger, the founder of Planned Parenthood, carried on this mission of disseminating the message of population control through her emphasis on cutting down the "production of its least desirable members" (Sanger cited in Franks, 2005, p. 12).

The interplay of imperialism and racist discourse implicit in the rationality of population control was well evident in the tenor of one of the first conferences on population control, an invitation-only "Conference on Population Problems" organized by John D. Rockefeller, and the precursor to the formation of the Population Council led by Rockefeller. Describing the discursive formulations that circulated in the meeting and specifically referring to the observations shared by Warren Weaver, the head of the natural sciences division of the Foundation, Connelly (2008, p. 157) observes:

> Warren Weaver . . . openly worried that development aid would only make Indians "nigger rich." Weaver translated: "a man who finds out that he has a little income—And what does he do? Well, at that moment he just stops working four days or a week, and he just sits there. I do not think this is what we want to bring to India."

Worth highlighting is the racist tone of the narrative that forms the bellwether of population control interventions. The racist depiction of the Indian body given to laziness is the site of the intervention.

Pointing to the discursive erasure that forms the basis of population control, Connelly (2008) further describes the meeting, "Indians were represented at this meeting, but they did not represent themselves. Instead, participants projected their prejudices onto the subcontinent as they speculated about its future. The only one who had actually published research on India, Kingsley Davis, had visited the country for the first time six months earlier." The power of the materiality of population control is also communicative. The depiction of the raced other as a threat and as incapable of agency is essential to the discursive distance from the sites of pronouncement and the power exerted over these sites. The colonial knowledge establishment establishes its hegemony precisely through its removal from the subject positions, prescribing, implementing, and evaluating interventions from a distance.

The gene pools of the global South emerged as targets of population control interventions, mediatized through the womb of the Third World woman that became the site of population control interventions. The fear of the fast-reproducing, illiterate, impoverished, superstitious, and colored masses from the underdeveloped world propelled the overarching eugenic vision guiding population control programs (Connelly, 2008). This narrative of controlling the reproduction of the masses that threaten civilization emerges as a consistent theme in the early population control establishment. Connelly (2008, p. 174), for instance, offers a correspondence authored by Margaret Sanger, the champion of population control as a solution to the world's problems:

> I consider that the world and almost our civilization for the next twenty-five years, is going to depend upon a simple, cheap, safe contraceptive to be used in poverty stricken slums, jungles and among the most ignorant people. I believe that now, immediately there should be national sterilization for certain dysgenic types of our population who

> are being encouraged to breed and would die out were the government not feeding them.

Eugenics forms the cornerstone of population control, voiced in the circulation of affect around the threat of a burgeoning population of the primitive forms of human life, marked as the sites of sterilization. These earliest notions of selectivity through directed control embodied the ideas of efficiency and effectiveness in curbing population growth. Those races and population segments would be selectively encouraged to reproduce that fit into the efficiency and growth logic, and those segments of the population that were seen as impoverished would be discouraged from reproducing as they are deemed unfit for reproduction. The collaboration among experts, funding agencies, and planners in the global North and the elite in the global South worked toward controlling the population threats that were discursively situated in the reproducing masses of the lower classes. Therefore, the racist logic of population control also played out class interests, serving the agendas of dominant power structures to deploy expert knowledge toward the agenda of consolidating, reproducing, and securing class power.

The narrative of population control emerged into a narrative of family planning alongside the early developments of neoliberalism based on the notion that creating opportunities for family planning enabled more efficient and effective economies, thus leading to development (Dutta, 2008; Rogers, 1962, 1973). Economic growth, the key marker of the neoliberal logic, was predicated on the logic of population control. Development in the Third World happened through economic growth, and economic growth was thought to be unleashed through the systematic control of population growth. The economic linkages of population control are evidenced in the positioning of population control within the ambits of WB.

Moving into the 1990s, the Washington Consensus reimagined the racist logic of eugenics by incorporating it within the language of rights and access, most visible under the reframing of population control as family planning. Population control has emerged under neoliberalism within the framework of reproductive choice and reproductive health, tied into corporate efforts, corporate social responsibility programs, and public–private partnerships. For instance, under the aegis of the "Profit Initiative," USAID has actively worked to redirect the blocked assets—profits generated by TNCs in developing nations that prohibit the transfer of money outside the nation—into population control programs. In 1992, USAID signed a $36.4 billion contract with the accounting firm Deloitte and Touche to act as a mediator for turning $200 billion in blocked assets into "private" contributions for family planning in the host countries (Mosher, 2008). As a part of the contract, the private corporations would get to claim a deduction on their tax returns as charitable deductions. Engaging the private sector in the broader agendas of family planning would also work toward minimizing the trade barriers for contraceptive commodities and promote the development of a regulatory framework promoting the expansion of private sector family planning products and services (Liagin, 1996).

Inherent in the neoliberal logic of family planning is the erasure of the voices of the women of the global South who are framed as audiences for empowerment. Family planning programs are presented as resources and capacities for empowerment, meeting the large "unmet need" of women globally, and yet in the articulation of the problem of population, the voices of the women are largely absent. Consider, for instance, the description of the USAID work on family planning on the website of the organization (www.usaid.gov/what-we-do/global-health/family-planning):

> More than 215 million women worldwide want to avoid pregnancy, but are not using a modern method of contraception. Enabling couples to determine whether, when and how often to have children is vital to safe motherhood and healthy families. Voluntary family planning has profound health, economic and social benefits for families and communities.

Note here the role filled in by USAID as the voice of women worldwide. The desires of the women for avoiding pregnancy are narrated through the expert voice of USAID, juxtaposed in the backdrop of the articulation of the absence of modern methods of contraception. The trope of modernity is articulated through the presentation of technologies of contraception as the much-needed solutions for women worldwide that are absent from the marketplaces of the global South. The language of empowerment is prescribed within this discursive space of absences. Technologies of contraception are tools of empowerment through access to which couples can become enabled consumers. The language of neoliberal governance shifts discursively to one of individual choice and voluntary family planning enabled through access to the technologies of contraception. Worth noting here in the empowerment-based logic of neoliberalism is the interpenetrating relationship between health and development, where family planning brings health benefits for the family constituted within the logics of economic welfare and progress.

The economics of population control is tied to the status quo logic of controlling populations that seemingly threaten the geosecurity of the dominant power structures. Economic development is married to health through the language of population control, later reframed as family planning. Population control, in other words, is seen as a mechanism for forging economic growth. Consider, for instance, the case made for increasing USAID funding for family planning programs by the former directors of the USAID's family planning program (Speidel, Sinding, Gillespie, Maguire, & Neuse, 2009):

> The United States once led the world in supporting access to affordable, high-quality family planning education and services for people in developing countries. In one of the great success stories of the modern era, women around the world now bear half as many children as their grandmothers did, contributing greatly to maternal and child health and global economic growth. USAID was instrumental in this achievement and in reducing the burden of poverty and disease worldwide. (p. 10)

The emphasis is placed on economic growth. Family planning is a link that connects health to global economic growth. Reducing population size is seen as a way of reducing poverty, oblivious to the largely unequal patterns in global distribution of resources underlying poverty. Worth noting, however, are the taken-for-granted assumptions. The emphasis on global health is shifted from raising questions of structural inequality and social justice to questions of population control, individualizing responsibility and simultaneously holding individuals and families accountable for their own growth, health, and development in a vastly unequal world. The development logic of population control continues to be reified in the neoliberal logic of family planning, albeit reframing top-down intervention strategies in the language of consumerism, client-driven interactions, and community participation.

Co-Opting Culture

Increasingly, for population control programs directed at the global South, cultural adaptation is an essential component. Culture, as a collection of shared values, offers guidance about the most effective strategies for developing persuasive messages. Coined as *cultural sensitivity*, this approach focuses on developing culturally relevant messages that are adaptive to the local culture. To adapt to the local culture is to develop messaging strategies that are aligned with cultural variables, thus enhancing the persuasive effectiveness of the targeted message. Note, for instance, the 2002 report issued by the Institute of Medicine, *Speaking of Health: Assessing Health Communication Strategies for Diverse Populations*, suggesting that "to maximize communication effectiveness, one should adapt message formats, sources, channels, and frequency of exposure for different audiences. Factors such as age, gender, race/ethnicity, and sexual orientation all draw on different interactions with the world and lead to different understandings regarding what is important and what is appropriate" (p. 56). Salient here is the emphasis on culture as difference that can then be incorporated into effective program delivery. Therefore, the effectiveness of top-down health interventions designed by experts is tied to the development of appropriate cultural categories to measure culture and then deploying these categories to deliver appropriately targeted messages. The prevailing diffusion of innovations framework maps out cultural characteristics that work as impediments to the diffusion of the innovation, embodying the racist narrative of development communication that labels culture as a primitive site, antithetical to the linear story of development and progress. Although now the racist language is now readjusted to a discourse of cultural sensitivity, the underlying prevailing logic is one of culture as a site of resistance to innovation that must be overcome through the cultural tailoring and targeting of messages.

The transition from early development communication to neoliberal articulations of development communication witnessed the emergence of new frameworks of social marketing, targeting, public–private partnerships, and community-based interventions that now shifted from the racist narrative of early development communication to a culturally sensitive narrative of development communication. Culture emerged as a category to be understood adequately so that it can be appropriately incorporated into the intervention. Consider the social marketing framework of family planning that identifies through formative research with target communities a variety of barriers to behavior change and then addresses these barriers through social marketing strategy. For instance, surveying a range of family planning programs across the globe, Smith (2005) notes that external and environmental factors such as religious opinions, husband's approval, and oppositions from members of reference groups are barriers to the adoption of family planning. Identifying these as pull factors, factors that are anti–behavior change, social marketers then work on ways to addressing the pull factors. In Bangladesh, campaign planners and program managers identified the influence of religious leaders as barriers to the adoption of family planning, thus beginning a serious effort to recruit the support of clerics to the campaign.

Similarly, Adeleye, Aldoory, and Parakoyi (2011) describe a culturally targeted family planning intervention that applies the framework of culture to engage men in Ekiadolor through a communication intervention to impact family planning. The understanding of the local culture offers a guiding framework for the development of communication strategies directed at men with the goal of increasing the adoption of family planning methods in the targeted community. Noting the role of culture as a variable that can be operationalized and measured, communication planners focus on deciphering the relevant cultural characteristics so that effective interventions can be developed. In the domain of new communication technologies for the diffusion of health-promoting behaviors, scholars suggest the valuable role played by cultures in shaping the understanding of the appropriate technology-driven intervention strategies (Ndiaye, 2014).

Empowerment as Disenfranchisement

Health communication as development has been refashioned under the language of empowerment in neoliberalism, repositioning population control programs in the language of family planning, and framing population control as individual-level health choices enacted through participation in the market. The racialized body of the postcolonial "other" emerges into the discursive spaces of neoliberal health communication interventions as a subject of empowerment, to be rewarded with the gift of power delivered by the intervention through the health commodities offered in the market. Empowerment, in this scenario, translates into giving power to a targeted subject population, albeit understood as the transformation of the subject into the participating consumer. The subject, as the target audience of health communication, must be given power through the communication intervention.

Intrinsic to the identity of the target is the absence of agency such that agency can be transferred through the expert-driven processes of empowerment, simultaneously locating the responsibility of health at the level of the individual. The experts hold the key to the appropriate messaging strategies that empower. Constructs such as self-efficacy and collective efficacy work as guiding principles for the development of messages. Consider, for instance, the discourse of community participation as empowerment within the context of family planning interventions defined in the ambits of adoption of family planning methods (Smith, Witte & Lazell, 2005). Here, *empowerment* is defined in terms of the community gaining the power to mobilize resources for disseminating the family planning intervention. Community norms defined in the ambits of social change are attached to predetermined campaign objectives shaped by development actors, university partners, and NGOs. In reporting on community norms in Nigeria, Smith et al. (2005) discuss community participation in the context of community norms, knowledge deficits, and community communication processes organized around HIV/AIDS. The notion of power in the ambits of enactment of positive health behaviors is crystallized in conceptualizations of self-efficacy and collective efficacy. Efficacy, conceptualized as the ability of the individual to enact her or his choices, is framed within the ambits of the family planning intervention.

Participation: The New Hegemony

Integral to the perpetuation of the neoliberal logic as the dominant logic of health communication is the ability of neoliberal governance to co-opt the language of participation to serve the top-down agendas of development agencies, IFIs, and TNCs. Neoliberalism achieves its hegemony through the language of participation, framing grassroots empowerment as the key to economic efficiency and growth, and simultaneously pushing this empowerment in narrowly consolidated frameworks of new technologies of control. The expert, on one hand, is integral to the neoliberal intervention as the developer of technologies and persuasive strategies, and he or she is simultaneously obfuscated in the language of bottom-up participation and grassroots-driven change. The veneer of participation itself becomes a tool for top-down dissemination, with the agenda already having been preconfigured by the power structures in the form of goal setting and objective development. The show of participation works in this case as a tool of co-optation that incorporates the community as a mechanism for the delivery of solutions.

The study of community participation processes through analyses of social network preferences, social network formation, and social network influences offer important insights to communication campaign planners (Boulay & Valente, 2005). Boulay and Valente (2005), for instance, discuss the ways in which the community social environment shapes the contraception choices of women. Studying the role of discussion networks in the context of contraception choices, the authors observe that adding a woman who is a contraceptive user to a discussion network is likely to increase the chances of contraceptive adoption. The community, understood in terms of community social networks, is seen as a site of influence, being incorporated into health communication as a means for increasing exposure to family planning information, family planning innovations, and social norms of contraceptive use. The community and participation in the community get defined in terms of social networks that promote the targeted behavior. Similarly, social capital, understood as community trust, community participation, and community satisfaction, is registered within the ambits of promoting the targeted health behavior, that is, contraceptive adoption. The community thus is a communication channel that serves the purpose of disseminating the proposed intervention designed by experts (Boulay, Storey & Sood, 2002).

Privatizing the Business of Population Control

An array of private sector organizations emerge in the context of global health with the goal of delivering population control interventions, albeit reconstituted under the rhetoric of family planning and increasing access to the market among the underserved sectors (Armand et al., 2007). The underserved sector is ontologically labeled as underserved in relationship to the presumed universal need for a health product, in this case, a family planning intervention delivered by the private sector. For many of these private sector organizations operating in the reproductive health sector, the commoditization of reproductive health lies at the heart of the business model. The delivery of health interventions is intrinsically linked with the creation of new markets for reproductive health products, captured in the social marketing language of untapped consumer needs and consumer demands. Communication is seen as the practice of creating consumer demands for health products.

The *Goli ki hamjoli* (Hindi for "Friends of the Pill") campaign, developed with the goal of increasing the demand for and use of commercially available oral contraceptives (OCs) among women in India, captures this intersection of private sector, development agencies, and population control (Leavell & Sinha, 2005). The campaign, funded under the Program for Advancement of Commercial Technology—Child and Reproductive Health (PATH-CRH) and the ICICI Bank, brought together India's largest private bank and the health and pharmaceutical industry to create large-scale market demand for OC products in the urban sectors in North India. Whereas PATH-RCH provided funding support for market expansion and demand creation as well as technical assistance for social marketing, ICICI provided financial oversight and industry networks with OC pharmaceutical partners. The campaign, developed by the creative agency Ogilvy and Mather, utilized the combination of public relations and advertising strategies to create market demand for OCs. In addition to nineteen theme and informational advertisements, the campaign deployed local volunteer activities through community leaders, networks of physicians to offer free counseling on reproductive health and low-dose OCs, physicians as spokespersons for the campaign, outreach to prospective consumers through NGOs, peer networks of satisfied OC users, referred to as *hamjolis* ("friends"), outreach to physicians through seminars, and outreach to indigenous systems of medicine practitioners (ISMPs) and pharmacists through hamjoli field representatives. The partnerships with pharmaceutical firms formed a key component of the campaign. The overall organizing structure of the campaign, launched alongside the neoliberal reforms being introduced in India, predicated the market as the site of delivery of health, defining the role of targeted advertising and public relations activities constituted within a social marketing framework in creating and sustaining consumer demand for a health product.

In addition to creating demands for existing products sold by private corporations, the business of population control is also tied to creation of new products such as female condoms. Investments therefore are made into new products addressing new needs in the market. Innovation, new technologies, and new solutions are tied to the creation of new market opportunities. For instance, the Bill and Melinda Gates Foundation (to be discussed in depth in Chapter Three) funds a number of technology-driven entrepreneurial solutions motivated by this emphasis on the market for reproductive health products. One such example is the Next Generation of Condoms grant call under the Grand Challenges Explorations initiative. The new generation of condoms funded through the initiative and brought to market through private partnerships addresses population control goals through the creation of new market demands. New needs and demands must be designed in order to capture the business potential of a market, simultaneously capturing the health needs of a consumer segment. The definition of health is intertwined with the commoditization of health, articulated in the creation of a market segment of untapped consumers who would deliver exploitable profits to the private sector. Consider, for instance, one such condom innovation, Origami condoms, supported by the Gates Foundation: "Our mission is to provide unique, pleasurable products that people enjoy using to increase consistent consumer uptake. Our unique, pleasure-oriented innovations may soon reshape the future landscape of the old rolled condom industry on a global scale" (www.origamicondoms.com/#!about/cwvh). The investment in the health innovation is tied to the creation of a new market, which in turn is codified in increased consumer uptake of the innovation.

Also, specifically in the realm of health communication, a number of these private organizations operating in the public relations and advertising sectors play out the role of developing communication strategies, creating tactical materials as well as providing evaluation research for population control programs. The role of the private sector is defined in relationship to the creation of strategic communication (promotional, publicity, events, and community relations) materials that would create the health need and subsequently push the health commodities directed at addressing these needs. In the introduction to the WB technical paper number 223, titled "Strategies for Family Planning," written by Piotrow, Treiman, Rimon, Yun, and Lozare (1994), Janet Merode, then director of the Population, Health, and Nutrition Department of the Bank, notes the intersection of economics and population control, "Institutional capacity to design, manage, and evaluate communication activities must be developed. The private sector, with its emphasis on entertainment and advanced technology, must be involved" (p. v). The private sector is incorporated into the logic of capacity building for population control.

The ascendance of the private logic of population control is accompanied by the hegemony of the managerial logic, supporting the political economy of an MBA-trained managerial class that is paid large percentages of program budgets to carry out these programs. Consider, for instance, the report issued by the Private Sector Advisory Facility Working Group of the Center for Global Development on the role of partnerships with the private sector in the health sector, highlighting the role of the private sector in contributing managerial and consulting skill sets that are otherwise not available in the public sector:

> By and large though, the biggest constraint is that policymakers and public officials in government agencies lack the technical know-how and management systems to engage the private health sector. Policies such as those related to contracting or accreditation, that engage and influence the private sector are complex and challenging. They require specialized skills and new practices built on experiences in other countries and basic principles of economics, regulation, business, and other fields. The technical assistance available to public officials in developing countries, however, typically offers little support and expertise on private-sector engagement. (Harding, 2009, xiii)

The hegemony of technical assistance is built upon the depiction of a need that is brought about through the universalized articulation of engagement with the private sector as a model for organizing health. Skill sets in management and accounting create opportunities for a new managerial class, operating in a new market segment of health and development, supposedly bringing together knowledge of economics, regulation, business, and other fields into development projects. Note here that these skill sets are articulated within an implicit and predetermined logic of private sector of engagement.

In the name of capacity building and technical assistance, new programs and market opportunities for the private sector are opened up for the training and professionalization of new managerial classes that offer the expertise and skill sets that are otherwise absent in the public sector. Central to the logic of private sector engagement is the depiction of the deficits in the public sector, constituted in relationship to an assumed logic of the greater effectiveness and efficiency of the private sector. In other words, intrinsic to the dominance of private sector organizing of health is the absence of capacities in the public sector, cyclically tied to predetermined objectives of private sector engagement as the assumed model of effective and efficient delivery of health.

On a similar note, healing relationships are redefined in terms of client-provider interactions (CPIs) that must be guided by individualized service delivery, shaping informed choices to be made by clients, respecting clients' rights to privacy, and two-way interaction with the client (Kim et al., 1992; Murphy & Gryboski, 2005). The framing of the health client constitutes health as a commodity in relationship to a service, also attaching articulations of service delivery to constructions of privatized choices. This framework of privatized health services delivery then creates the market for health communication and health management experts who offer the professional guidance on effective CPI, which is further tied to the adoption of family planning methods. The language of two-way communication plays a pivotal organizing role in creating a market for communication trainers, managers, and professionals who can then provide the training in relevant communication skills to the provider and the client with the goal of enabling dialogue. Dialogue in this sense is very much constituted within the logic of privatized control and creation of new markets for both communicative capital and commoditized health products and services.

Health, Agriculture, and Food Insecurity

Another dominant theme of development that played out in the earliest communication work was embodied in the diffusion of agricultural technologies, rooted in the Cold War narrative that diffusing agricultural technologies in the Third World would solve problems of global hunger in the decolonized Third World and would thus minimize the security threat to the "free world" posed by communism and revolutionary movements of the dispossessed (Holt-Gimenez & Patel, 2009). Based on the framework that the lack of access to food was produced by the absence of appropriate agricultural technologies, solutions were devised in the form of technological solutions that needed to be diffused in the targeted Third World.

The role of communication therefore was conceived in the form of disseminating the message of agricultural technologies in agrarian communities, forming the bulwark of early diffusion of innovations campaigns. USAID, in collaboration with universities and research stations located in the global North, played a key role in the dissemination of expert-driven agricultural innovations, with nation-states and research centers in the global South serving as mechanisms for diffusing the innovations. The technologies therefore embodied expert knowledge rooted in the North and were driven by the assumption that experts knew better the best solutions to agriculture in the Third World, juxtaposed against the backdrop of recipient local communities in the global South that practiced primitive agriculture. The primitive–modern binary circulated in fundamental expressions of development, reiterating the expert knowledge of the Western/Northern expert juxtaposed against the backdrop of the local farming practices. The transition from development interventions to neoliberal interventions was shaped by the large-scale corporatization of agriculture starting in the 1970s, with a shift into global policy interventions that promoted the diffusion of privatized agricultural technologies. The role of development agencies such as USAID was reconfigured in pushing interventions that fostered new markets for U.S. TNCs.

Agricultural Technologies as Modernization

As noted in the introduction to this section, the agenda of global development was shaped by the ideology that the introduction of new agricultural technologies would address global poverty and hunger, and would in turn, therefore, build spaces of support for U.S. foreign policy, simultaneously halting the spread of communism in the global South (Cullather, 2010). Agricultural technology was a weapon in the fight against communism. With access to basic food and forms of livelihood, the global poor would not be participating in transformative revolutions. Social change thus defined was understood as the dissemination of agricultural technology. The green revolution narrative was quintessential to the top-down dissemination of agricultural innovations from the global North, primarily the United States to the nation-states of the global South, namely, India, Pakistan, the Philippines, and Mexico. Communication, formulated under the framework of diffusion of innovations, was integral to the strategic dissemination of messages targeting to induce behavior change in the targeted populations.

A study with hybrid seed corn diffusion conducted by Ryan and Gross (1943) in two rural Iowa communities offered the foundation of the diffusion of innovations scholarship, itself an innovation in the social sciences that accompanied the innovations in agriculture funded by USAID, reflecting a broader climate of Cold War investment in agriculture and social sciences as strategies for creating security and promoting growth in the Third World. The observation made by Ryan and Gross (1943) that the adoption rate of the hybrid seed corn followed an S-shaped pattern over time offered the basis of the diffusion of innovations framework (Rogers, 1995; Rogers & Svenning, 1969). The S-shaped adoption curve, attributed to the different categories of farmers in the target community, sparked social scientific work on identifying target categories of farmers and developing appropriate messaging strategies. The innovators were more cosmopolitan and owned larger farms than the later adopters did, and early adopters were more likely to hear about the hybrid seed corn from the salesmen, while later adopters heard about the innovation from their neighbors. Developing appropriate segmentation strategies based on the diffusion curve became the basis for the development of appropriate communicative strategies (Rogers, 1983, 1995).

The U.S. Department of Agriculture harvested the knowledge gained from early diffusion of innovation work for spreading the adoption of new agricultural technologies among the rural sectors of the globe (Rogers, 1983, 1995). Rogers (1995) eloquently pointed out that the diffusion of innovation studies were critical landmarks in speeding up the diffusion process of agricultural revolutions, thus bringing modernization and the promises of higher productivity. Celebrating the miracles of the diffusion of innovations model, he wrote:

> Thanks to Ryan and Gross (1943), the rural sociologists had an appropriate paradigm to guide their diffusion studies. Thanks to the agricultural revolution of the 1950s, these diffusion scholars were in the right place (state university's colleges of agriculture) at the right time. The result was a proliferation of diffusion studies by the rural sociology tradition: 185 by 1960, 648 by 1970, and 791 by 1981. (1995, p. 56)

The successful diffusion of innovation studies were subsequently extended to the developing nations of Latin America, Africa, and Asia (Rogers, 1971, 1995). The U.S. government saw it as a tool for expanding U.S.-style modernity across the globe (Rogers, 1983).

Sponsored by USAID and several private foundations, diffusion programs focused on spreading agricultural innovations such as seeds, agricultural equipment, and fertilizers to the Third World (Rogers, 1995). Technology occupies center stage in the neoliberal narrative of agriculture, constructing agriculture as the domain of profiteering. The green revolution narrative emerges into the discursive sites of neoliberalism as a mechanism for expanding into new markets in new spaces. The neoliberal desires of the United States work hand in hand with the neoliberal imaginaries mapped out by agro-corporations, funding agencies, and foundations, formulating, for instance, new spaces in the African continent as new sites for the neoliberal experiment in technology-driven agriculture.

Structural Adjustment Programs

The United States, through its powerful role in shaping the Washington Consensus, has catalyzed a climate of global agricultural trade reforms to foster markets for U.S.-based TNCs. The WB has played a key role in global transformations through the SAPs. The SAPs have served as instruments for creating new markets for transnational seed companies, exerting pressure on Third World nations to open up their markets (Shiva & Bedi, 2002). The transition from peasant-based systems of agriculture to systems of agriculture that were largely dependent on agro-chemical and seed corporations has been shaped by a narrative of development that promises greater agricultural productivity to questions of hunger.

WB has been instrumental in pushing for structural adjustment through its loan programs that were directed at making the national seed industries more market responsive (Shiva & Jafri, 2003; Shiva et al., 2002). The privatization of the seed sector has fostered large-scale profit extraction for TNCs on the basis of the sale of monoculture seeds accompanied by the sale of fertilizers, pesticides, and agriculture machineries. The locally situated community-based organizing frameworks of seed sharing have been replaced by commoditized purchase of genetically modified seeds manufactured by TNCs. Government-sponsored extension programs initially created demands for seeds among indigenous farmers and then privatized the seeds in the realm of the market.

Claims of increased efficiency, optimization of pest resistance, and generation of maximum yield serve as the interpretive frames that seek to disseminate GM seeds among farmers. These GM seeds respond to fertilizers and pesticides, which are also manufactured by the TNCs, thus leading to an external input-driven system as opposed to the traditional system that was driven by internal inputs in local agriculture. Also, farmer's cropping patterns have shifted from mixed cultivations to monocultures of hybrids that are pushed by external inputs, turning agriculture into monolithic spaces framed in the language of the market. The emphasis on privatization has also influenced the types of loans available to farmers, shifting from public sector low-interest loans to high-interest private sector loans (Shiva, 2002). Overall, then, the political economy of agriculture has shifted from traditionally sustainable local forms of agriculture to commoditized forms of large-scale capitalist agriculture brought under the control of TNCs through the displacement of the subaltern sectors from their access to forms of livelihood.

Simultaneously, the emphasis on external liberalization of agriculture has dictated that agricultural subsidies be reduced, which has resulted in the price rise of foodgrains supplied through the Public Distribution System (PDS). The price rise of the foodgrains supplied through the PDS then led to the rise in the market prices of foodgrains. In order to address the underserved sectors, the government introduced a specifically subsidized PDS. However, the subsidized products typically do not reach the underserved markets and are leaked into other areas because of the intertwined relationship between power structures and distribution mechanisms.

Trade, Tariffs, and Agreements

Trade liberalization, one of the early instruments of neoliberal globalization, was constituted in the formation of GATT in the postwar era (Dutta, 2011). Depicting the global flows of power, GATT symbolized the hegemonic leadership of the United States in pushing global policy formulations that opened up new opportunities for U.S.-based TNCs even as the U.S. private interests enjoyed tremendous protections during the early growth years. The specific objectives of the United States in negotiating the GATT were constituted in the relationship of the U.S. state as an instrument of pushing new markets for U.S.-based TNCs (Hudec, 1988). Developing countries struggled to protect their infant-industries and to gain special status in the international trade market (Hudec, 1988; Madeley, 1999, 2000). Power and access to structures of decision making played pivotal organizing roles in constituting the uneven terrains of implementation of GATT such that the United States continued to protect sectors of U.S. agriculture even as it worked through GATT to push for developing countries to open up their markets.

The Agreement on Agriculture (AoA) came into effect in 1994 as a result of the 1986–94 Uruguay Round of the GATT, subjecting agricultural commodities to the multilateral trading rules (Gonzalez, 2002).The agreement obliged participating nations to provide market access to other nations and to significantly reduce traditionally allowed domestic supports and export subsidies to farmers. Depicting the power inequities that constituted the terrain of contestation, the AoA was shaped by the intense rivalry between the United States and the European Union (EU) for world agricultural markets, and developing countries were almost entirely left out of the negotiating processes. As a result, the AoA served only to institutionalize the existing inequities between developed and developing countries by restricting policy options available to developing countries to promote food security; the agreement enabled developed countries to continue to subsidize and protect domestic producers while requiring developing countries to open up their markets to foreign competition.

The erasure of food security as a criterion of decision making in the AoA has had negative repercussions for small farmers who have limited infrastructures for addressing the needs for these farmers both in terms of agricultural policies and in terms of other public services. Furthermore, the principles of liberalization in agriculture have focused on the logic of competitiveness, based on the argument that a nation can increase its efficiency by producing and exporting commodities in which it is relatively efficient and by importing commodities in which it is relatively inefficient (Shiva, 2002). However, Shiva (2002) demonstrates that the comparative advantage for countries actually turns into absolute advantage for TNCs because as a nation starts importing large quantities of a particular commodity on the basis of the very logic that the commodity is cheaper on the international market, the international prices go up because of the large-scale import possibilities.

Agreement on Trade-Related Aspects of Intellectual Property Rights (TRIPS)

TRIPS defined a powerful moment in constructing globally a relationship among knowledge, profiteering, and trade, coming into effect in 1995 as a result of the 1986–94 Uruguay Round of the GATT (Peet, 2003). Privileging the protection of innovations as an organizing framework for interpretation, the WTO positioned TRIPS as protecting the right of innovators to prevent others from using their innovations and the right to negotiate payment from others in return for using their innovations. *Intellectual property* is defined in terms of the following organizing concepts: copyright and related rights (the rights of performers, producers of sound recordings, and broadcasting organizations); trademarks; geographical indications, including appellations of origin; industrial designs; patents, including the protection of new varieties of plants; the layout—designs of integrated circuits; and undisclosed information (Peet, 2003).

Particularly worth noting in the context of agriculture is the organizing logic of ownership of nature within private structures (Shiva, 2005, 2007, 2010). Privileging a definition of innovations that reiterates the development narrative of conquest of nature is tied to the privatized logic of neoliberalism, constructing biology as a site of profiteering (Shiva, 1988, 1991). Patents created new opportunities for capitalizing genetic resources, turning seeds as resources for profiteering and catalyzing the rapid growth of the biotech industry. The birth of biocapital is a productive moment of neoliberalism, fostering growth in the private bio sector as catalyst for economic growth (Sundar Rajan, 2006). According to Sunder Rajan (p. 3), "Life sciences represent a new face, and new phase, of capitalism and . . . biotechnology is a form of enterprise inextricable from contemporary capitalism." The bioeconomy is intertwined with the speculative financial economy, with the biological becoming the source of profit generation through the privatization of the biological under the ambits of TRIPS. The communicative inversion deployed by TRIPS, as elsewhere, centers on the powerful role of the U.S. state in creating new markets for U.S. TNC-based biological innovations, albeit under the rhetoric of free trade and private enterprise.

The interpretation of what knowledge is, how it will be measured, and whom it will benefit is constituted in a capitalist logic, and this is exemplified in TRIPS as an instrument of neoliberalism. The capitalist logic reflected in TRIPS is colonial in its deployment of symbolic and material processes of colonialism that historically extracted vast resources from colonies to fuel the industrial revolution. The biopiracy of basmati in South Asia reflects this very colonial strategy, reconfigured as the primary organizing instrument of global biocolonialism. The communicative inversions of knowledge claims to serve biocapitalism is embodied in the business model of RiceTec, a Texas-based multinational agro-company that patented basmati rice, deploying the power of legal processes that promote such piracy. Basmati rice is traditional to India and Pakistan, and in 1997 comprised 4 percent of India's export earnings, securing premium prices in the international market. In September 1997, RiceTec successfully applied for several patents on the basmati rice and grain lines. The Pakistani and Indian governments refuted the patents, stating that the plant varieties and grains already exist as a staple in India, and that neither variety of rice can be grown in the United States. The U.S. Patent and Trademark Office rescinded fifteen of the twenty patents granted. However, the five remaining patents continue to permit RiceTec to exclude others from making, using, and selling its patented basmati rice in the United States until September 2017, limiting the access to the international market among the rice-producing nations in South Asia where the knowledge of basmati is grounded.

RiceTec's U.S. patent claimed the invention of "novel rice lines with plants that are semi-dwarf in stature, substantially photoperiod-insensitive and high-yielding, and that produce rice grains having characteristics similar or superior to those of good quality basmati rice grains produced in India and Pakistan" (Trade and Environment Database [TED], 1998).

However, the policy does not take into account that the patent takes ownership of genetic material originally developed by South Asian farmers; the germplasms from these varieties were initially collected in the Indian subcontinent and later deposited and processed in the United States and other places. Add to that, TRIPS also allows the patent holder to usurp the "basmati" name, which itself could jeopardize the sale of basmati from South Asia owing to confusion (TED, 1998).

The TRIPS agreement threatens food security not only by not recognizing indigenous community's rights over their resources but also by enabling biopiracy or the appropriation of local biological resources without consulting the local community or representative state actors. Constituted in the realm of questions of legitimacy of knowledge structures and the political economy of these structures, TRIPS treats indigenous knowledge as common property because it is not patented; the idea here is that if knowledge is not patented, it is not owned and therefore is open to technological modifications, which can then be patented (Bodekar, 2003; Woods, 2002). Woods (2002) and Bodekar (2003) note that the TRIPS agreement does not extend either patent or geographic protection to the traditional knowledge of indigenous people; for example, the patent laws under TRIPS do not adequately recognize traditional form of breeding as "prior art" (that is, the entire body of knowledge available to the public before a given filing or priority date for any patent, utility model, or industrial design). This has thus led to multinational biotechnological corporations successfully seeking patents on foodgrains (Woods, 2002), which in turn negatively impacts local economies. In addition, TRIPS enables biopiracy to take place with relative ease, especially in less-developed countries that are rich in genetic resources and low in technology. Access to technology in developed countries allows richer countries to harness and reproduce genetic material for patenting, thereby enabling the expropriation of local resources and bringing them under the instruments of control of TNCs to generate greater global profit.

The patenting of food grains can have major implications for the economy and food security in the least-developed countries (LDCs). In many of the LDCs, foodgrains such as rice form a vital part of people's diet. According to Owens (2002, as cited in Woods, 2002), Asian rice provides up to 85 percent of the calories in the daily diet of 2.7 billion people. According to TED (1998), with the basmati patent rights, RiceTec will be able to not only call its aromatic rice basmati within the United States but also label it basmati for its exports. This means farmers that depend on basmati cultivation and export in India and Pakistan will not only lose out on the 45,000-tonne U.S. import market, which forms 10 percent of the total basmati exports, but will also lose their position in markets like the EU, the UK, the Middle East, and West Asia. This would certainly hit the local economy in rice-growing regions of India and Pakistan. As farmers lose markets for their crops, their incomes will be hit hard, leading to increased inability to spend on a basic necessity like food. Thus, the very resources that are a part of the day-to-day life of indigenous groups have to be purchased at a price from the technologically advanced countries and from TNCs, creating the scenario for continuous exploitation.

The combination of TRIPS and SAPs in the context of the Third World has resulted in the large-scale co-optation of agricultural spaces as the markets for the seeds and chemicals manufactured by TNCs. Furthermore, TRIPS emerges as a disciplinary site of control for enacting the hegemony of global agribusiness such as Monsanto. With 94 percent of the global acreage for genetically modified food in 2000 under the control of Monsanto, for instance, large sectors of agricultural land come under the purviews of Monsanto, thus ensuring that the TNC uses the articulations of intellectual property rights to bring additional acres of land under its domain and further establish its dominance in global markets. As local farmers are surrounded by more and more genetically modified seeds in their agricultural lands, the chances of contamination with genetically modified seeds increase, and so do the threats of being litigated by the agribusiness giants for the violation of property rights.

The threat of litigation for violating patent laws operates as a site for hegemonic control of agriculture, bringing additional agricultural lands under the purviews of TNCs. For instance, Monsanto sends inspectors into farmlands, investigating the crops and trying to find some of its patented crops; if these patented crops are found not to have been purchased directly from Monsanto, the farmers are threatened with lawsuits (see Dutta, 2013). With the pollution of farms with Monsanto seeds, which can be carried by wind, non-Monsanto farmers can be sued for violating the intellectual property rights of Monsanto. The violence of biocolonial capitalism is deployed through the claims to knowledge, the privatized ownership of knowledge, and the deployment of knowledge to serve monopoly structures of capitalist control. Patenting works as an instrument of biocolonialism.

Corporatization of Agriculture

With the advent of neoliberal interventions in agriculture, agriculture turned into a capitalist mode of profiteering, accomplished through the implementation of agricultural technologies as mechanisms for extracting maximum profit through the processes of dissemination of agriculture. Innovations in biotechnology funded by the state were turned into profitable products that could be further developed by agricultural transnational corporations such as Monsanto and Syngenta. Development continued to be at the forefront of reconfiguring agriculture, now in the form of privatization processes that privileged rich farmers with large landholdings mostly producing crops to feed into the corporatized agro-structure.

Corporatization of agriculture followed the technology-driven restructuring of agriculture. The introduction of miracle seeds, fertilizers, pesticides, and other agricultural technologies into the peasant sectors of the Third World created markets for agro-TNCs that produce these seeds, fertilizers, pesticides, and technologies, also turning agriculture into a site of profiteering. Thus a new market was created in the agro-business sector for the global agro-businesses, primarily situated in the United States and UK. Development therefore was important to the creation of new markets for hegemonic agribusinesses, offering entry points for transnational corporations into Third World spaces, driven by the logic that primitive local agriculture was ill equipped to address the local food needs. As we will see in the section on the nature of evidence making, much of the claims on the effectiveness of innovations in addressing global poverty and hunger were often missing. The communication theorists working on the diffusion processes focused on building the science of persuasion underlying the assumed universal solutions without really interrogating the scientific viability of these solutions or without really calling for evidence on the effectiveness of the proposed innovations.

The neoliberal transformation of agriculture has also resulted in new forms of dependence on global market volatilities. Encouraged by structural adjustment programs pushed by IFIs, as farmers have shifted from growing food crops to growing cash crops in the quest for economic growth, their ability to secure food has become dependent upon the economic performance of their crops in the international market (Narayan & Petesch, 2002; Shiva, 2000, 2002, 2005). Whereas traditionally farmers participated in agriculture sustainably and grew a wide variety of crops that were often grown in rotation in order to feed themselves and their families, neoliberal agriculture pushed farmers into global market cycles, commodity trading, and speculation. As demonstrated with the monoculture crop failures in various parts of the globe, the neoliberal organizing of agriculture has made farmers more vulnerable to global market trends and to the performance of their crops in the international market, thus also making these farmers food insecure (Shiva, 2000, 2002, 2005). In the context of large numbers of farmers who have gone into major debt to invest in technology-intensive commercialized agriculture, suicide emerges as a response to the cycles of debt, thus threatening human health in its most fundamental form.

Agriculture, Commodities Market, and Speculation

With the bursts in the technology and housing bubbles in the mid-2000s, financial investors started investing heavily in the commodities market. Commodities futures are standardized legal agreements between two parties to transact in a physical commodity at a particular designated time in the future, thus guaranteeing a given price for both producers and consumers. Speculators in the commodities market generate profits on the basis of speculations on the rise or fall of prices of commodities in the future. As the food prices started rising in 2005–6 as a result of climate-change-related drought patterns, the shift to agro-fuel-based agriculture, the rise in oil prices, and the rise in industrial meat production, speculators started investing heavily in the commodities market, with little or no regulation from the government. The profits to be secured in the agricultural commodities sector also resulted in "crossovers," with banks crossing over to financial instruments such as commodities, agribusinesses developing investment arms, and commodities traders crossing over into financial markets. The constitution of agriculture within the realm of speculative capitalism rendered it volatile, intrinsically tied to profit, and alienated from questions of food production, local needs, and sustainable processes.

The Hegemony of Science and Knowledge Production

Development communication efforts are driven by the expert-driven production of knowledge that identify target communities that need the innovative technologies of development. The large-scale reorganization of global agriculture has been brought about through the language of science that is intrinsic to the diffusion of innovations framework. The benefits of scientific innovations are assumed by the proponents of the framework, framing critical interrogations and calls for evidence as antiscience (Shermer, 2013). The language of science in this sense works to promote and perpetuate structural inequalities in communicative access. Communicative inequality plays out in demarcating the possibilities of participation in knowledge-producing structures. While scientific experts produce knowledge about the green revolution and its effectiveness, local communities and local community experience are erased. Against the backdrop of the techno-deterministic framework of development pushed by communication practitioners, the knowledge of local communities itself becomes the site of intervention, to be transformed through persuasively framed communicative strategies. The hegemony of science is reproduced through the communicative inequalities embodied in development and neoliberal discourses. The role of the communicator is constituted in creating persuasive top-down messages, appropriately framed through the scientific knowledge of communicative effectiveness, to achieve desired goals predetermined by the collusion of science, technology, and development sectors. Discursive spaces for conversation and dialogue on the basis of the consideration of wide-ranging evidence and experiences are erased.

Erasure of Evidence

The narrative of the "green revolution" maps onto the global organizing of agriculture a techno-deterministic framework promoting seeds, pesticides, fertilizers, irrigation technologies, and agricultural machineries as miracles of development (see the speech delivered by then USAID director William Gaud to the Society for Development in 1968; he coined the term *green revolution*). The coinage of the term *green revolution* served as a branding strategy for technologically driven agriculture, suggesting a peaceful revolution in raising communities out of poverty and in feeding the hungry in the global South, as opposed to a "red revolution" (Cullather, 2010, p. 233). The green revolution stood in for and symbolized miraculous developments in agricultural productivity induced by new technologies, accompanied by abundance displacing hunger.

With the rhetoric of the "green revolution" offered as a magic bullet of development, it is worth interrogating the evidence regarding the effects of the green revolution. In 1968, the year that the term *green revolution* was engineered, India, Turkey, Philippines, and Pakistan, four of the countries where high-yield varieties of seeds were introduced, demonstrated phenomenal crop yields. These crop yields were positioned alongside agriculture biotechnology as the panacea to global food insecurity and inaccess.

The ideology of technology-driven globalization is built on the circulation of words, images, and messages that frame the universal success of the promoted technologies. The narrative of the "green revolution" is reworked into a neoliberal imagination of "Green Revolution 2.0 (GR 2.0)" (Cullather, 2010). The technological determinism of the development establishment and its later neoliberal incarnations is captured in the idea of the magic bullet, which is seen to bring the miracle of development and progress to the underserved sectors of the globe, thus lifting them out of poverty. Integral to this narrative is the powerful role of top-down communication as a public relations tool, framing the messages of technological innovation, countering public opinion, and winning over the antiscience opponents. Communication is integral to the legitimizing processes of establishing the hegemony of the techno-deterministic solution of the green revolution. This billion-dollar public relations industry works through its media relations, community relations, and lobbying activities to circulate the rhetoric of uncharted progress, almost always devoid of or contradictory to the evidence on hand. When alternative evidence is indeed presented, the public relations industry works aggressively to delegitimize such evidence or to label it as antiscience.

Development Actors

The global hegemony of neoliberalism has been achieved and continued to be exerted through the globally connected networks of power, embodying particular relationships of organizing that serve the interests of capital. Global structures such as WHO; international financial institutions such as WB, WTO, and IMF; global development agencies such as USAID and DfiD;

private corporations; nation-states; NGOs and foundations; and local elites work hand in hand in constructing a global structure of health governance that is driven by expertise, the commoditization of health, the privileging of the private sector and the simultaneous erasure of local knowledge, local participatory processes, and local democratic possibilities that interrogate the global restructuring of health. A health communication framework that interrogates the meanings of health and the communicative processes that constitute health depicts that the neoliberal organizing of health.

World Health Organization (WHO)

Starting in the 1970s, WHO started coming under criticism from the United States because of its emphasis on building public health infrastructures and social services. The United States pulled its funding from WHO and started establishing its role in shaping the global health agenda through funding directed toward WB (to be discussed in the next section). As WHO sought to reinvent itself in the context of global neoliberal reforms, it adopted the language of privatization as a response to global health issues.

As WHO calibrated its ideology along the lines of WB and other IFIs, the WHO framework started pushing for the privatization of health. Public–private partnerships emerged as key structures for the delivery of health and health care, spearheading the privatization of public health resources. Erased from the discursive spaces of WHO are critical interrogations of the structural logics of privatization of health and the health consequences of these logics, especially as they relate to social determinants of health.

This fundamental contradiction in the WHO logic that, on one hand, makes notes of structural determinants of health and, on the other hand, proposes private sector solutions is perhaps best exemplified in the recommendations proposed by the WHO Commission on Social Determinants of Health (CSDH) (WHO, 2008) in the report titled *Closing the Gap in a Generation: Health Equity through Action on the Social Determinants of Health*. The report articulates the role of the private sector in strengthening accountability and in investing in research and development in diseases of poverty. Suggesting that the private sector has great potential, the CSDH report locates accountability in the hands of private actors:

> Recognize and respond accountably to international agreements, standards, and codes of employment practice; ensure employment and working conditions are fair for men and women; reduce and eradicate child labour, and ensure compliance with occupation health and safety standards; support educational and vocational training opportunities as part of employment conditions, with special emphasis on

> opportunities for women; and ensure private sector activities and services (such as production and patenting of life-saving medicines, provision of health insurance schemes) contribute to and do not undermine health equity. (p. 45)

Note the realm of accountability shifted into the hands of the private sector and the simultaneous absence of workers, labor organizations, popular grassroots organizing, and activists in the grass roots who exist outside the realm of the dominant framework of the civil society.

Accountability as understood from the framework of WHO is constituted in the responsible behavior of the private sector in ensuring fair working conditions, supporting opportunities for improving worker productivity, and directing private sector activities such as in the pharmaceutical and insurance sectors toward health equity. Erased from the discursive space are questions of accountability of the corporate sector to state structures and to grassroots participatory spaces. The role of the civil society is constructed in the narrowly defined realm of social determinants of health policy planning, programs, evaluation, and monitoring, removed from the realm of holding the private sector accountable. The roles of international organizations such as the multilateral specialist and financial agencies are formulated in terms of holding recipient governments accountable using health equity and social determinants of health indicators. The agenda of WHO itself is defined in terms of guiding policy coherence, supporting measurement and evaluation, and building internal WHO capacity.

The market-driven logic circulated by WHO is reflected in its use of communication in the communication-for-behavioral-impact (COMBI) programs (Renganathan et al., 2005). COMBI draws upon the Alma Ata declaration of WHO to combine the social mobilization component of WHO programs with directed behavior change strategies drawn from the principles of social marketing. The program adds an element of social mobilization to the social marketing model, shaping integrated marketing communication strategies through sequential elements of market assessment, situational market analysis, and objective setting directed at individual behavior change. Essential to the definitional terrain of COMBI is the definition of the citizen as a health consumer to be targeted through effective integrated marketing communication (IMC) messages promoting behavior change:

> An integrated and coordinated approach with credibility is vital. Integration does not occur at the level of the agency or of the media. Integration takes place with consumers; therefore, IMC *begins with the consumer*. (Renganathan et al., 2005)

The mix of communication channels, including interpersonal counseling, point of service promotion, advertising, community mobilization, and political mobilization, are shaped by appropriate behavioral objectives determined by planners on the basis of marketing principles.

The effectiveness of COMBI in achieving directed behavior change is correlated with effective planning and market assessment, establishing behavioral goals, establishing political commitment among political leaders and bureaucrats, organizational adaptation, and collaboration with local communication management expertise in the private sector in the form of advertising and public relations organizations. The vital role played by the private sector in delivering an effective social marketing strategy is highlighted by Renganathan et al. (2005, p. 317): "Advertising agencies bring a refreshing creativity to program design and implementation as well as the opportunity to mobilize new private sector partners drawn from the client-base of advertising agencies that deal with the commercial world."

World Bank (WB)

WB played a key role in shaping the global transformation of the health care sector. The SAPs introduced across Latin America in the 1980s, for instance, weakened public infrastructures, destabilized the welfare state, and eroded social services such as health care (Muntaner et al., 2006). Particularly under attack were services that were directed at the poor, turning these services into privatized resources. The SAPs weakened the public sectors by draining resources away from them, contributing to the deterioration in quality of health services as well as resulting in inefficiency within public health sectors. These inefficiencies in the public health sectors then were turned into justifications for WB interventions in the arena of health. In 1993, WB (Peet, 2003) issued *The World Development Report: Investing in Health*, marking the direct entry of WB into the health arena, replacing the role of WHO through the powerful backing of the United States (discussed in the previous section), and offering the overarching logic for the restructuring of health care as a privatized commodity, managed through insurance companies, health management organizations, and transnationals in the financial, banking, and investment sectors (Waitzkin, 2011). In Mexico, WB sponsored reforms in the health care and pension components of the social security system (Waitzkin, 2011).

WB introduced concepts such as disability-adjusted life years (DALY) to measure the effectiveness of interventions. DALY quickly became the hegemonic standard for the evaluation of health systems and health programs, reducing human beings into effective and productive labor. Moreover, the very framework of DALY constituted the categorization of human beings into productive and unproductive groups, thereby directing resources toward restoring the health of productive groups of the population that promised to contribute to the economy.

Beyond the programs directly directed at health through the restructuring of health care, health became integral to the rhetoric of WB, realized through its mantra of poverty alleviation. Global restructuring programs were framed in the language of poverty reduction since the 1970s, with an explicit shift to poverty reduction in 2000 onward. WB used structural adjustment programs as tools for alleviating poverty, paradoxically leading to further marginalization of the poor and consolidation of resources in the hands of the power elite.

Projects such as microcredit (MC) are celebrated as models of grassroots-driven bottom-up development, with WB playing a leadership role in pushing the MC model of development. The WHO report submitted by the CSDH (WHO, 2008), *Closing the Gap in a Generation: Health Equity through Action on Social Determinants of Health*, celebrates the MC model as an organizing framework for creating better health among the poor by lifting people out of poverty. The language of entrepreneurship and self-reliance places ownership of economic growth in the hands of the poor, framed in the language of empowerment and turning the power into new markets for the investment, finance, banking, telecommunications, technology, and consumer goods sectors. However, as depicted through the example of the Grameen Bank (GB) in Bangladesh, celebrated by WB and its neoliberal ideologues as a model of grassroots-driven development, the grassroots-driven model of development among the poor becomes a mechanism for extending the reach of transnational capital to this sector, now defined as a new consumer market (Muhammad, 2009). As noted in this section and in the previous section, the agendas of WB and IMF are intertwined with the powerful role of development agencies, and particularly USAID in shaping global development agendas along the lines of U.S. transnational corporate interests.

International Development Agencies

Since World War II, international development agencies emerged as major powers in pushing top-down ideologies of political and economic organizing through the narrative of development. The global dominance of free market capitalism can be tied to the hegemonic functions of development agencies such as USAID and DfiD. Through their development programs in family planning, agricultural development, and economic restructuring, these dominant development actors pushed the U.S.-centric notions of free market capitalism. For instance, the economic agendas of development programs are deeply embedded within logics of population control and are simultaneously married to development interventions directed at opening up countries to TNCs. The goal of development is married to the strategic role played by the state (in this case the United States and UK) in opening up new markets.

Health is framed as a commodity, and the goal of communication is seen as a functional vehicle for generating demands in new markets. Take, for instance, the notion of demand generation articulated in the Health Communication Capacity Collaborative funded by USAID (Health Communication Capacity Collaborative, n.d.): "The Demand Generation Implementation Kit, the 'I-Kit,' is a step-by-step guide to developing communication strategies to increase demand for nine priority commodities, and provides cross-cutting tools, guidance and adaptable commodity-specific content." The goal of health communication is interpreted as a framework for generating demand for health products as commodities. Here is an additional description of the strategies for demand generation. Demand generation increases awareness of and demand for health products or services among a particular intended audience through social and behavior change communication (SBCC) and social marketing techniques. Demand generation can occur in three ways:

1. Creating new users—convincing members of the intended audience to adopt new behaviors, products, or services
2. Increasing demand among existing users—convincing current users to increase or sustain the practice of the promoted behavior and/or to increase or sustain the use of promoted products and services
3. Taking market share from competing behaviors (e.g., convincing caregivers to seek health care immediately, instead of not seeking care until their health situation has severely deteriorated or has been compromised) and products or services (e.g., convincing caregivers to use oral rehydration solution (ORS) and zinc instead of other anti-diarrhea medicines)

Note here the notion of demand generation as an overarching framework for addressing development-based health communication. The role of communication is constituted within the structure of the market, as a tool for generating user demands within the market. The language of market segmentation and consumer behavior are deployed to offer a framework for approaching demand generation.

Demand generation programs, when well designed and implemented, can help countries reach the goal of increased utilization of the commodities by:

- Creating informed and voluntary demand for health commodities and services
- Helping health care providers and clients interact with each other in an effective manner
- Shifting social and cultural norms that can influence individual and collective behavior related to commodity uptake
- Encouraging correct and appropriate use of commodities by individuals and service providers alike

The goal of communication is constituted around shaping community cultural norms and encouraging individual behavior (Storey & Figueroa, 2012). Demand for the commodity is generated through messages and symbols that perform the persuasive function. As we will witness throughout the book, persuasion emerges as the prevailing structure for interpreting and framing health communication within the neoliberal landscape.

Development investments thus offer the facade for performing public relations functions for TNCs, simultaneously exerting the power of development funds to shape economic policies in targeted nation-states. The concept of health diplomacy, for instance, tied to the narrative of development is embedded within this broader structure of profiteering and generating business opportunities. The investments made by USAID in development interventions as well as in global structures of knowledge production on health interventions colonizes knowledge of health interventions. Putting forth a neoliberal model of health, development agencies such as USAID frame health in the language of the market, tied to economic productivity and participation of the labor force in economic activities. USAID invests into structures such as the Health Communication Capacity Collaborative as a global structure for shaping the global discourse of health communication and health promotion. The language of capacity building is co-opted within the neoliberal structure of development programming to create a global repository of development knowledge constituted in the dominant notions of development, health, privatization, free market, and commoditization. Consider the following depiction of the collaborative (Health Communication Capacity Collaborative, n.d.):

> Strengthening the capacity of local organizations is at the heart of HC3. The project focuses on three levels: organizational, individual and national. HC3 supports skills strengthening for a wide variety of audiences, including program managers, journalists, video and radio producers, health workers and counselors, health education units and local government staff. At the national level, HC3 can help local governments and key implementing partners design, update, or

> implement national health communication strategies to better coordinate ongoing efforts. HC3 will also engage a variety of partners including the private sector, the media and universities. HC3 is compiling health communication tools and approaches that have proven successful or are believed to be promising and innovative. When complete, this collection will be assessed and distilled into a widely shared toolkit of health communication best practices to help increase and sustain capacity.

The language of best practices, capacity building on health communication knowledge, and skills training are constituted within the broader USAID-funded agendas of family planning. Health communication capacities, understood narrowly in relationship to articulations of the market, are framed within the language of growth and productivity. The global leadership offered by USAID frames and constrains the global language of health communication within the ambits of participation in the market, market mechanisms, and individualized consumption.

Structures of knowledge production such as Cornell University and Johns Hopkins University, through large funding resources deployed by USAID, emerge as the sites for articulation of truth, creating neutral-sounding knowledge claims. Appeals to science and scientific knowledge manufactured from these sites work to circulate specific agendas of development framed within these broader structures constituted by USAID. For instance, the corporatization of agriculture through the language of biotechnology as a solution for the green revolution is given a public face through the dominant structures of universities. Often obfuscated from USAID funded partnerships, for instance, are the profit-making goals of private actors or the profits that are generated for TNCs from the production, circulation, and dissemination of public knowledge. The development structure is a key player in serving the neoliberal agendas of transnational capitalism.

Third World Elites, Nation-States, and NGOs

The ability of the neoliberal framework to perpetuate itself as the dominant frame of health communication targeting the Third World is intrinsically connected to the ability of the framework to recruit Third World elites, both from within the nation-states as well as from diaspora populations as carriers of the development logic. Third World elites occupying dominant class positions within nation-states align themselves with global funding agencies and international financial institutions to diffuse the threats of revolution through population control and agricultural biotechnology. To the extent that these Third World elites are represented in the neoliberal network of health communication campaigns, the campaigns can claim to have evolved from the early culturally insensitive developmentalist logics to culturally sensitive interventions designed by multicultural and diverse planners and programmers representing the Third World spaces where the culturally sensitive campaigns are being run. Such tokenism then rests precisely on the logic of representation, where the co-optation of the local elite from the margins is intrinsic to the co-optation of the margins as the subject of intervention. The career of these Third World postcolonial subjects/academics/experts (myself included, as someone trained in U.S. institutions and hired and funded by U.S.-based institutions) is tied to their ability to parrot the language of development and sing the songs of technologically mediated progress, albeit couched in the language of cultural sensitivity, culturally meaningfulness, Third World participation, and diversity promotion.

Private Sector

As depicted throughout this chapter, the private sector is a key player in the context of health, both with reference to its health-depleting effects that need to be regulated and also with its direct roles in the health sector through the privatization of health products and services as sites of profiteering (more on the private sector in Chapter Four). Insurance industries and health management organizations are constituted around the speculation, management, evaluation, and assessment of risk. Transnational corporations in the health sector include pharmaceutical companies, manufacturers of health technologies, biotechnology companies (both in the food and medicine production sectors), banks, financial institutions, managed care organizations, and several communication and marketing organizations that carry out often publicly funded interventions on health issues. The profit margins of the privatized enterprises is established through development solutions pushed by international development agencies, establishing new markets and arenas of health innovations under the umbrella of development. In the communication sector, private organizations delivering social marketing solutions emerge as key actors in the delivery of health interventions.

The neoliberal organizing structures of health communication incorporate the private sector into the realm of development, thus aligning the private sector within the development narrative rather than as a departure from this narrative. The private sector is portrayed as bringing in specific managerial strategies, knowledge, and expertise in order to serve the health needs that are traditionally conceived of as operating within the development arena. The privatization of health therefore transforms health into a site of profiteering in the global landscape. The logic of the private sector is driven by profits secured from transactions in markets. To the extent that profits drive market-based health solutions, these solutions then are packaged as solutions of development for the global South. Private–public partnerships offer the chador for the deployment of privatization in the development sector, operating in a variety of health sectors.

Development: Ideology and Evidence

A central argument of this book draws the relationship between development and privatization under neoliberal organizing. Neoliberal organizing centers meaning on poverty alleviation through the dissemination of privatized commodities and through expert-led technological innovations, continuing the thread of expert-led social change embodied in development organizing. Neoliberalism, on one hand, embodies the ideology of expert-led development solutions prescribed in the form of technological fixes, and, on the other hand, promises participation and entrepreneurship as solutions to resource inaccess. The neoliberal ideology of development is marked by its roots in top-down communication that is not borne out by evidence, simultaneously deploying the rhetoric of scientific modernity to disseminate neoliberal governance across global spaces. As is evident throughout the chapter, the networks of powerful Western states (the United States and UK, in the form of their development agencies as well as in the form of military interventions) play key roles in shaping the global development discourse.

Power is both distributed in networks as well as consolidated in geographically concentrated centers. In this sense, neoliberalism can be best described as a pseudoscience that has captured the imagination of the social sciences through its very appeal to science. Ironically, neoliberalism is founded on a spirit of anti-evidence and information inequality while at the same time it uses this language of evidence, accountability, and transparency to consolidate power in the hands of transnational capital. Claims of economic growth facilitated by neoliberal policies are not borne out by evidence. Strong claims of development that suggest that neoliberal growth would lead to trickle-down growth, for instance, are not supported by the large-scale impoverishment we witness among the poorer sectors of the globe. Communication plays a powerful role as an instrument of spinning, in managing messages through persuasion and framing. The literatures in science communication and health communication privilege studies of framing, embedded in the notions of effective persuasive effects of specific framed messages. Instead of fostering transparent spaces for information equality where spaces of access are created to nurture debate, communication framed as persuasion is directed at silencing dissent by framing such dissent as antiscience. The role of communication is one of manipulation and control rather than one of enabling democratic participation and dialogue in discussions of benefits, effectiveness, costs, side effects, and alternatives.

A large proportion of the communication literature, rooted in the origins of the discipline in World War II propaganda research and in the propaganda work of spin masters such as Edward Bernays, examines the ways in which persuasion can be catalyzed to achieve desired objectives conceived by powerful actors funding communication projects, and catalyzes communication as a persuasive magic bullet. Absent from the discursive spaces of communication are serious questions regarding the nature of risks, effects, effectiveness, and so on. Absent are questions of fostering democratic spaces for discussions and debates on evidence on effectiveness, side effects, and limitations. Active agendas, often mired in conflicts of interest, are deployed to serve the agendas of transnational power structures, with organized efforts of discrediting alternative voices that raise critical questions. Questions of uncertainty and probability that are intrinsic to the processes of science are replaced by persuasive agendas that target behavior change in the forms of family planning, promotion of new vaccines, and promotion of technologies such as mammography, presented in a language of certainty (Bertrand, Babalola & Skinner, 2012).

The disdain for the participatory capacity of everyday people becomes evident in the celebration of top-down expertise that flows through Cold War social sciences, where knowledge flows from the centers of expertise in the global North to the recipients of the intervention in the Third World. Academic spaces of knowledge production located in the North are vital to this discursive inequality. Reproducing the communicative inequality in legitimating the political economy of global health work, and more specifically global health communication work couched in the language of development, the dominant structures of knowledge position the Third World as incapable of knowledge production. Knowledge is a powerful instrument in the reproduction of communicative inequalities, determining who can and cannot participate in discursive spaces and simultaneously deploying the content claims made by knowledge structures toward profitable goals. Development structures such as USAID play powerful roles in shaping the discursive terrain of knowledge through their funding of interventions situated within the liberal framing of health as individualized consumer participation. Knowledge of interventions in reports, briefs, journal articles, and so on, make up the body of knowledge on development communication.

Appeals to science are discursively circulated to foreclose participatory possibilities of interrogation rooted in the lived experiences of communities. For instance, situating the large-scale farmer suicides against the backdrop of the massive conversion of farming into Bt. technology-driven farming and the inequities in access to food that are reproduced by technology-driven agriculture, the scientific establishment deploys the narrative of science to frame critical questions as antiscience (see, for instance, the op-ed published by the scientist Nina Federoff in the *New York Times* on August 8, 2011, and the piece on the liberal war on science by Michael Schermer published in the *Scientific American* in 2013). The progressive narrative of science as universal and beyond the realm of interrogation erase democratic possibilities for discussion of evidence, knowledge claims, side effects and unintended effects, and conflicts of interest. For instance, what are the ethical consequences when much of the efficacy and side effects testing of genetically modified crops is conducted by scientists paid by transnational agrochemical corporations selling the genetically modified crops and profiting from these sales? What are the possibilities of democratic citizen participation in science as science gets increasingly concentrated in the hands of the power elite, tied to corporate structures and global funding flows, and as science communication is relegated to a public relations function with the agenda of persuading target audiences through targeted framing of messages?

As noted earlier throughout the chapter, the language of participation is co-opted into the mainstream structures of development and health to facilitate the dissemination of top-down interventions based on expert knowledge. Participation is understood as a channel for dissemination that will secure buy in and sustainability for the intervention. Neoliberal health organizing catalyzes the expert-driven knowledge production processes inherent in Cold War development communication, further turning this knowledge into a commodity that extracts profits through public–private partnerships, commoditization of health, and market-driven sale of expert products. Creating the need for the health product in the global South is essential to the building of markets for TNCs that profit through the privatization of the "bio."

Discussion

This chapter attends to the ways in which development discourse and development structures are integral to the global hegemony of neoliberalism. The production of development knowledge framed within liberal interpretations of health has historically connected health to growth, economic development, and modernization achieved through the adoption of new technologies (such as birth control technologies and agricultural technologies). The large-scale push for these technologies in target countries has facilitated new markets for transnational capital, accomplished under the language of development. Development, narrowly defined as the adoption of innovations and new technologies, is therefore intrinsically connected to the creation of new markets as sites of profiteering. Universities, intervention teams, and civil society organizations have worked hand in hand with private corporations to circulate the prevailing neoliberal definition of health as a commodity.

CHAPTER THREE

FOUNDATIONS AS NEOLIBERAL INTERVENTIONS

The mandate for health is increasingly being set by global foundations that have taken up the discursive sites of policy making and program planning through their ability to secure access to financial resources and to deploy these resources to shape health policies and health programs. Access to economic resources emerges as the determiner of policy textures and policy structures globally, thus leaving dramatic capacities of influence in the hands of foundations. With budgets that are larger than many nation-states, these foundations play key roles in shaping the global policy agendas and in running programs that displace state-run health programs. The elite-driven framework of neoliberalism where experts configure through top-down decision making the nature of problems and the corresponding nature of solutions becomes evident in the force exerted by foundations in shaping the landscape of health policy making and programming (Plehwe, 2008).

The powerful role of foundations in establishing the neoliberal agenda is evident in the emergence of institutions such as IEA, Center for Policy Studies, and the Adam Smith Institute in the United States and AEI, Heritage Foundation, Cato Institute, Hoover Institution, and Manhattan Institute in the UK (George, 1997). With annual budgets running in millions of dollars funded by foundations such as the Ford Foundation, Bradley Foundation, Coors, and Mellon, these institutions played the pivotal roles of marketing neoliberal ideas. This chapter examines closely the role played by foundations globally in structuring health as a private enterprise. The chapter will work through the interplays of power and knowledge within the ambits of the role of foundations in shaping health-organizing structures across the globe.

Power, Foundations, and Knowledge

Since the early years of development communication, foundations played powerful roles as the public face of private interests in shaping the landscape of public policy. Historically, the Rockefeller Foundation played a defining role in shaping policy frameworks and intervention design, guiding the

Neoliberal Health Organizing by Mohan J. Dutta, pp. 91–110.

frames around the identification of problems and the creation of corresponding solutions, especially within the broader domains of development and health solutions. These foundations offered funding into development programs often carried out by NGOs, with collaborations with academic structures as experts in the production and dissemination of knowledge. For instance, the agenda of population control as the defining parameters of health and development communication work emerged through the early work of the Rockefeller Foundation, identifying population control as a key global problem, connecting it to the underlying logic of capitalism, promoting free markets, and ascertaining the geosecurity of the dominant nation-states.

The powerful role of foundations in shaping global health agendas has been accelerated and intensely magnified under neoliberalism, turning social problems to the domain of capitalism, as the site of action for those very same capitalist structures that lie at the heart of these global social problems (Dutta, 2011; Fauboin, Paige & Pearson, 2011). These processes of privatization of the global health agenda are well evident in the rapid increase in private funding for global health, from 19 percent in 1998 to 26.7 percent in 2007 (Ravishankar et al., 2009).

"Philanthrocapitalism," a term capturing this marriage of philanthropy and capitalism, emerges on the global stage as the logic for privatizing problems such as poverty, poor health, and inaccess to resources, presenting as a solution the very organizing structures of capitalism that reproduce the problems of poverty, health inequalities, and poor health outcomes. Social problems are interpreted through the language of the market, often defined as the lack of access to the market, and therefore offering further commoditizing as the solution to problems of poverty, inequality, and health inaccess. The privatization of these problems therefore becomes the organizing logic of philanthrocapitalism, turning these social problems into new markets for capital, creating new market opportunities, and circulating the discourse of "win-win relationships" to consolidate the power of contemporary capitalism. This logic of privatization is well captured in the following articulation by the performer activist Bono in an interview given by Bono and Bill Gates at the Forbes 400 summit on philanthropy at the United Nations, New York (Lane, 2013):

> What was shocking for me as an activist was to learn how important the role of commerce was in ending extreme poverty and the role that entrepreneurial capitalism has played in taking people out of extreme poverty. Right now capitalism is in the dark. It's on trial. There's a sense of the "us" and "them," the 99 percent, the 1 percent, those who've gamed the situation, those who've been screwed by the situation. Some

> of these accusations, of course, are ridiculously far-fetched. But some of them are not. It's critical that [entrepreneurial philanthropy] somehow coheres in the 21st century into a new sort of shape and form. What I learned from Bill and Melinda is that it wasn't just going to be their cash that would be put to work but that the most important thing that they would contribute would be their brainpower.

Philanthrocapitalism then is seen as the powerful role of commerce in ending extreme poverty. The role of entrepreneurial capitalism is seen as one of utilizing the logics of entrepreneurship to address problems of poverty. The privileging of the managerial narrative of capitalism in working toward solving global problems is married to the portrayal of the fundamental problems of capitalism as extreme. Rather than create opportunities for structural transformation, the logic of philanthrocapitalism works to further consolidate resources in the hands of global capital.

Power reflects the positions of access to structures of decision making, resource allocation, policy development, program implementation, and evaluation. Power is directly intertwined with access to structures of capital, creating points of leverage for shaping global policies. In this scenario, foundations not only shape policies by directing the movement of resources, but they are also integral to the formations of knowledge around the problems of global health.

Foundations work precisely to undermine the regulatory climate, proposing global solutions that are not accountable to democratically elected state structures, and create additional unregulated markets for TNCs. Popular democracy and state formations are therefore seen as barriers to the free flow of capital, framed in the language of efficiency, ineffectiveness, and lack of performance. Regulations, additionally, are often seen as barriers to the efficient and effective delivery of health solutions to key problems. The state therefore is portrayed as a barrier to the development of solutions that would work. The language of freedom and liberty are deployed simultaneously to create unregulated spaces for private operation, appealing to interpretive frames of efficiency to consolidate the global hegemony of neoliberal health organizing.

The Bill and Melinda Gates Foundation

The Gates Foundation has played a global leadership role in reshaping the contours of health within the agendas of neoliberal interventionism. The hegemony of the Gates Foundation is reflected not only in the monetary resources in global health controlled by the foundation but also in the power exerted by the foundation in shaping global health governance. Through its various funding initiatives, the foundation has inserted neoliberal meanings of health systems organizing conceptualized in terms of the privatization of resources, ownership of individual responsibility, and logics of efficiency as the bases for organizing health.

The entry of Gates into the global health scenario has generated positive impacts on the issues of access to health care and treatment; however, it has simultaneously generated large-scale public health problems by draining resources from existing public health programs and resources, from state-run infrastructures, and from basic health capacities in communities in the global South. Empowerment, individual responsibility, ownership, and participation emerge as buzzwords in the interpretive frames circulated by the foundation in its various projects, turning health into a product of individual choice.

Empowerment as a Neoliberal Trope

Empowerment is an organizing feature of neoliberal health organizing. The language of empowerment is essential to the placing of the responsibility on the individual, based on the prevailing belief that the empowered individual will help herself or himself. Through their emphasis on the language of empowerment, foundations have played vital roles in establishing the hegemony of neoliberal organizing in global health, while at the same time weakening public health infrastructures. Even as individuals are supposedly empowered through foundation-funded projects, communities are increasingly disenfranchised from their points of access to the basic forms of health care.

Consider, for instance, the "Contraceptives Are Not Controversial" campaign run by the Bill and Melinda Gates Foundation. The campaign is framed as a social change initiative, with a signature pledge page that states (www.no-controversy.com/):

> There is no controversy in empowering women to decide if and when to have a child. Today, more than 200 million women and girls in developing countries who don't want to get pregnant lack access to contraceptives. I believe every girl and woman deserves the opportunity to determine her future.

The campaign assumes for itself the expert position of one who does the empowering. Empowerment is constituted in the language of choice, the meaning of empowerment therefore understood in the liberation of the woman in deciding if and when to have a child. Note in the above excerpt the co-optation of local participation and structural access within the neoliberal framework of population control, albeit couched under the language of choice. The opportunity for girls and women in developing countries to have a choice is framed within the dominant frame of the Gates Foundation that constitutes poverty alleviation within the logic of population control. Missing, for instance, is the lack of access to fundamental resources such as food, clothing, and shelter that are often articulated in the voices of women in the global South. Empowerment of women is seen in terms of controlling population, reformulating it in the language of access and opportunity.

More important, absent from the articulation are the voices of the women from the developing world. The effectiveness of the top-down expert-driven logic of the foundation lies precisely in its ability to speak for the women of the developing countries, determining for them what resources they desire access to. The market logic of "want" and "need" are determined through the expert lens of the foundation and its organizing frame of contraception as a poverty-alleviation strategy. Web participants are given the opportunity to interact with the site by putting down their names and addresses and clicking on the pledge of support, thus turning the question of health care access into the trope of individual participation.

Technology-Centric Design Solutions

The solutions proposed by the Gates Foundation emphasize the dissemination of new technologies to problems of health, narrowly conceiving health solutions within the domains of innovation, invention, and discovery of new technologies. The product-driven monopoly economy promoted and leveraged by Microsoft emerges as the framework for reorganizing health, with an emphasis on constructing health solutions as new products, tied to the creation of new markets for transnational capital. Markets are tied to health needs, leveraging the delivery of services to low-income populations as a market for generating profits. The attractiveness of social change processes for private partners lies precisely in the profit-generating function of these processes. At the heart of the neoliberal ideology promoted by the foundation is this market fundamentalism, thus also capturing the technologically driven fantasies of the foundation.

The emphasis, therefore, is on the creation of specific technologies that would address the problems at hand. For instance, in its malaria program, the foundation puts emphasis on creating new technologies that would control disease-transmitting mosquitoes. Presenting the strategy overview for malaria control, the program description depicts the challenge, the opportunity, the strategy, and the areas of focus, turning malaria prevention into a management function and drawing upon lessons of the private sector. The technology of malaria control complements the managerial technology of needs assessment and strategy development. Under the title of "New Approaches for the Interrogation of Anti-Malarial Compounds" is the following:

> The goal of this topic is to support unconventional and radically new approaches, methods, and assays to analyze, characterize and prioritize anti-malarial compounds and to glean more information required for the development of next generation malaria drugs. We wish to encourage researchers to develop and apply innovative biological, chemical, computational, and systems-based approaches for the interrogation of anti-malarial compounds to maximize knowledge gained from the publicly-available anti-malarial compound set, and facilitate compound selection and development. Many of the proposed approaches might have broad applications in drug discovery, and we encourage researchers to harness emerging tools and approaches for the goals of this topic, and to apply innovative thinking so that new methods can be brought to bear on the needs of the developing world. (Gates Foundation, 2012)

Drug discovery and development are tied to markets, creating new tools, approaches, and methods to address the needs of the developing world. The next generation of innovations is positioned at the intersections of biological, chemical, computational, and systems-based approaches. The developing world in the global South is positioned as the new market for these innovations, the needs of which need to be addressed through the innovative technologies.

Another example of the technology-driven product-centrism of the Gates Foundation is the "Next Generation" condom challenge, working toward finding new solutions for HIV/AIDS prevention. The next-generation products that the foundation invests in are seen as potential solutions that would work toward preventing the spread of HIV/AIDS and reducing the incidence of unplanned pregnancies. For instance, the air-infused female condoms, an innovation funded by the "Next Generation" call, are seen as providing a new and effective birth control and HIV protection solution for women. Innovations in this sense are married to the continued promise of new markets. Note also the twin goals of family planning and HIV prevention that are brought together under the umbrella of the "Next Generation" funding, with both being framed as key challenges in global health.

In describing the "Next Generation" challenge, Sow and Ward (2013) point to "great ideas that could eventually address the need for new condoms that men and women will actually want to use." The generation of new ideas is intertwined with the quintessential "need" being positioned in new ways so as to generate "want" among the consumer segment. The commoditization of health is achieved through the promise of new markets for the innovations that are funded by the foundation. Product improvement becomes the underlying logic that captures into new wants and unexplored market demands. The development of the innovation is captured in the logic of the market, married to prototype testing, marketing, and distribution functions (see Gates Foundation, 2013a):

> Condoms have been in use for about 400 years yet they have undergone very little technological improvement in the past 50 years. The primary improvement has been the use of latex as the primary material and quality control measures which allow for quality testing of each individual condom. Material science and our understanding of neurobiology has undergone revolutionary transformation in the last decade yet that knowledge has not been applied to improve the product attributes of one of the most ubiquitous and potentially underutilized products on earth. New concept designs with new materials can be prototyped and tested quickly. Large-scale human clinical trials are not required. Manufacturing capacity, marketing, and distribution channels are already in place.

Concept design, prototype development, and quick testing offer the managerial logic for the development and sale of new products. Specific areas for innovation development are guided by parameters established by the foundation.

> We are looking for a **Next Generation Condom** that significantly preserves or enhances pleasure, in order to improve uptake and regular use. Additional concepts that might increase uptake include attributes that increase ease-of-use for male and female condoms, for example better packaging or designs that are easier to properly apply. In addition, attributes that address and overcome cultural barriers are also desired. (Gates Foundation, 2013a)

Attributes such as ease of use, preserving and enhancing pleasure, and ease of application define the characteristics of the innovation, seen as characteristics that are likely to improve uptake and regular use. Moreover, innovation attributes are depicted in cultural terms as addressing and overcoming cultural barriers.

One of the grantors funded by the "Grand Challenges Explorations Grants" is the Origami Enterprise, highlighted in the March 18, 2013, blog post "Reinventing the Condom" as an "an excellent example of a private enterprise focused on new condom design to promote consistent use by emphasizing the sexual experience" (Gates Foundation, 2013b). The Origami Enterprise defines its business model as "Radical New Condoms for the Twenty-First Century," captured in the tagline "Condoms Reinvented." Note here the use of the word *radical* within the context of new condom technologies that would appeal to new markets. The enterprise of social change works through the radicalness of innovations that create new demands and tap into hitherto untapped markets. The innovation of the Origami condoms is juxtaposed against the backdrop of the traditional condom.

> Our mission is to provide unique, pleasurable products that people enjoy using to increase consistent consumer uptake. Our unique, pleasure-oriented innovations may soon reshape the future landscape of the old rolled condom industry on a global scale. Rolled condoms were first introduced around 1902, just a year before the Wright Brothers' first successful flight at Kitty Hawk, NC. Airplane technology has advanced us to landing on the moon and Mars while the rolled condom has essentially remained the same. Today, over 100 years later, condom technology has now advanced with radically re-designed ideas, new materials, and significant functional changes for the 21st century. (www.origamicondoms.com/#!about/cwvh)

The advances in condom technology are constituted amid pleasure-oriented innovations that are seen to increase consumer intake. The promotion of the condom is tied to a market for the innovations, a consumer-defined unfulfilled need, and the openings for change driven by the innovation. The logic of the market as quintessential to the innovation processes is well captured in the following articulation under the title "Vaccine Delivery: Strategy Overview":

> Along with supply and demand, price is a critical element in the successful launch and sustainable use of any new vaccine. Without a clear idea of the demand for a vaccine and how it might be delivered, manufacturers have little incentive to invest in product development and manufacturing. We are addressing this challenge by working with private industry on innovative, market-based financing mechanisms to ensure that vaccines are developed at the lowest possible cost. (http://www.gatesfoundation.org/What-We-Do/Global-Development/Vaccine-Delivery)

Market-based financing mechanisms are married to the development of the innovation, voiced in the language of demand, investment, incentive, and cost.

The technology-driven fetish of the foundation is well captured in the following critique offered by Faubion, Page, and Pearson (2011, p. 217):

> The Gates Foundation draws much of its funding from the personal wealth of Bill and Melinda Gates, money that was made via the technology sector, specifically from Microsoft. This has arguably translated into a confidence in technology and "magic bullets" as solutions to health problems, a pathway which Bill Gates himself has publicly championed. It is clear that the preferences of the individual in this case have informed the work of the Gates Foundation, and have found natural allies in a global biomedical community and its counterpart firms. It is no surprise then that the Gates Foundation's disbursements have also augmented the natural bias toward biomedical solutions favored by many GHPs, whose vertical disease-specific programmes are often based on the deployment of specific vaccines, therapies, or drugs.

The meanings of health circulated through the power exerted by the foundation "scientize" and "sanitize" health (ibid.), turning it into a depoliticized problem removed from questions of building basic public health infrastructures, shaping social determinants of health, and building equitable basic health structures where health services and care are universally available. The biomedical fix circulated by the foundation, on one hand, privileges corporate powers, and, on the other hand, obfuscates questions of structural equity, redistribution of resources, and social justice.

Expertise, Top-Down Management, and Accountability

The management of the Gates Foundation embodies the technical rationality of expert-driven solution making, turning health-based decisions as managerial decisions based upon the lessons of corporate models of management. Teams of management consultants and MBA-educated midlevel managers are deployed to carry out projects, often disconnected from the local context and untrained in the broader public health, communication, and cultural complexities of local needs. The vertical structure of Gates projects ensures the top-down dissemination of power in projects that are conceived by the foundation, with measures of accountability situated within the structures of power in the foundation. This centering of expertise lies at the heart of neoliberal market reforms carried out globally, with power being transferred to the hands of experts in creating and sustaining global free markets. The early rise of neoliberalism was intrinsically tied to the powerful role played by experts and this continues to be reified in the global restructuring of health, as evident in the agendas of the Gates Foundation. The ideology of expertise continues to deploy expertise-driven solutions of health irrespective of the empirical evidence base that interrogates the value of this expertise-driven model.

Given the influence of the foundation in shaping the landscape of global health and especially so in the global South, the power of the foundation is played out in top-down policy and program interventions that are defined by technical rationality, simultaneously erasing processes of accountability to states, public bodies, citizens, or actors outside the opaque foundation structure. The appeal of technical rationality is circulated in its broader base in knowledge and expertise as opposed to the democratic and public processes of decision making in government-funded structures, which are framed as being political. In other words, the politics of the foundation is played out in its framing as apolitical, the hegemony of expertise (McCoy & McGoey, 2011). Thus, the very ideology of the foundation achieves its hegemony through the discursive portrayal of an ideology-free facade that is fundamental to the ideological and political pursuits built into the power of expertise (McCoy & McGoey, 2011). The organizational structure of the foundation offers a revolving door for powerful actors in the pharmaceutical, food and beverage, and agro industries, thus raising key questions regarding the processes of flow of power.

Most Gates projects are strictly controlled by the foundation, with management teams serving as core teams of designers, implementers, and evaluators, and running the projects in the parlance of corporate management. The foundation invests large sums of money in developing managerial resources and in hiring core expert teams to carry out the projects. These teams of experts receive disproportionate proportion of grant budgets, spending most of their time at centralized locations developing project plans, receiving data points through reports, and managing through these data points and through teams of experts within the managerial structures of projects. The expert teams are put together through top-down processes of selection, playing centralized roles at distant locales that are far removed from the lived experiences at the margins (Flock, 2009). For instance, for running the $100 million "Avahan" (meaning "call to action") campaign in India, the foundation hired the McKinsey consultant Ashok Alexander, paying him an annual package of $424,894 (Flock, 2009). The foundation recruited leaders from the private sector to fill its top management with the goal of implementing a business model of health promotion and dissemination (Flock, 2009). Absent from the centralized structures of "Avahan" are local communities of truck drivers, sex workers, transgender participants, and men who have sex with men, who are targeted as the recipients of the interventions.

Some of the recipients of Gates Foundation funding are entirely funded by the foundation, thus raising questions about the functions and roles of these organizations and the extent to which their agendas and operating processes are owned by the foundation. The NGO Program for Appropriate Technology for Health (PATH), for instance, came under heavy scrutiny in India for leveraging its NGO structure to field-test human papillomavirus (HPV) vaccines through a Gates Foundation–funded project (Kumar & Butler, 2013). The program was positioned by PATH as an observational study of HPV vaccines manufactured by GlaxoSmithKline, Merck, and Dohme, while it was in fact a large safety trial (Alliance for Human Research Protection, 2011). The government of India canceled the field trials under observations that the trials did not adequately include informed consent processes, failed to secure consent, and did not adequately monitor and report adverse events, which included the deaths of seven vaccinated children (see Dutta, 2013a). Particularly important are the roles of the Gates Foundation and PATH in seeking to push the vaccines into India's government-funded universal immunization program, thus also creating pathways for profits for the pharmaceutical manufacturers of the vaccines. Furthermore, worth noting is the conflict of interest in this case generated by the investment structures of the Gates Foundation and Gates' personal wealth in Berkshire Hathaway, which in turn invests a significant portion of money in GlaxoSmithKline, the manufacturer of the HPV vaccine pushed by PATH in India (McCoy, Chand & Sridhar 2009; Stuckler, Basu & McKee, 2011). Another HPV vaccine pushed by PATH in India is manufactured by Merck, which also is part of the Gates investment portfolio.

Close interrogation of the projects funded by the Gates Foundation, the decision-making processes and the evaluative structures, draws attention to the erasure of local voices from the discursive spaces. Communities that are identified as poor or underserved are targeted through Gates-funded work as recipients of programs, with strong surveillance, top-down directives, and minimal opportunities to participate in decision-making processes. More broadly, evident in the structure of the foundation is the absence of NGOs and activists from the global South, which are typically positioned as collaborators in disseminating top-down programs conceived by the foundation. Even in instances where the foundation leverages the participatory rhetoric to carry out its programs, participation becomes a co-optive tool to serve the agendas of foundation-funded projects.

Also absent are state and democratically elected structures of decision making, thus reorganizing local public health spaces on the basis of the agendas of the foundation simply by virtue of the extensive access of the foundation to capital. The absence of state and democratically elected processes from foundation-driven interventions sometimes leads to the weakening of state public health infrastructures, diversion of valuable state resources to foundation-driven agendas, and unstainable projects that are driven by episodic inflow of money. The problem of sustainability is particularly critical when local, state, and national governments have not been adequately involved, leading to short-term projects that leave behind large gaps when the project funding ceases. Add to the top-down processes the business-driven model of programming that is pushed by the foundation, and critical problems are created locally. For instance, in the backdrop of the Avahan campaign funded by the Gates Foundation in India, local social change projects started experiencing a dearth of volunteer peer leaders as the foundation started paying money to peer leaders to attract them. At the end of the project, many of these peer leaders who had taken to spending most of their time working on paid grant work found themselves in situations where the payments were no longer available. The NGOs working locally found themselves in changed cultural contexts of peer leadership where peer leaders expected to get paid after having worked on the Gates-funded campaign.

Economic Flows

The flow of power is tied to the access to economic resources in the hands of the foundation and the ways in which these resources are circulated in global networks of capital, reframed in the narrative of development. As noted earlier in Chapters One and Two, development therefore emerges as the trope for consolidating power in the hands of global capital. In the case of the Gates Foundation, the flow of economic resources depicts the marriage between the capitalist agendas of the foundation and the ways in which these agendas are accomplished through a narrative of development. For instance, the foundation promotes innovations in pharmaceutical technology development and in disseminating of pharmaceutical commodities in the global South, while at the same time it invests large proportions of its money in shares in the very same pharmaceutical corporations whose products it disseminates.

> Many of the Foundation's pharmaceutical development grants may benefit leading pharmaceutical companies such as Merck and GlaxoSmithKline, for example, via partnerships to test pneumonia and rotavirus vaccines (such as the ROTATEQ partnership and the Merck Vaccines network partnership with the Global Alliance for Vaccines and Immunizations network), experimental malaria vaccines (through Medicines for Malaria Venture, an NGO), cervical cancer

> vaccines (through PATH, an NGO, and Merck's vaccine Gardasil), and HIV interventions (through the Africa Comprehensive HIV/AIDS partnership). Johnson & Johnson has entered a clinical partnership to develop new HIV-prevention technology, noting "the work between Johnson & Johnson and the Gates Foundation is a strong, strategic, comprehensive relationship." (Stuckler, Basu & McKee, 2011, p. 6)

In these instances, the foundation becomes the face of the pharmaceutical TNCs, utilizing its philanthropic front to secure access to states and state structures, turning public spaces into private markets, and fostering new markets for the private corporations with which the foundation is intertwined.

The power exerted by the foundation therefore becomes a space for uncritical access of the foundation to development policies and programs, which in turn are turned into profitable spaces for private interests. In the example shared above, the private investments of the foundation directly and indirectly through Berkshire Hathaway into the pharmaceutical TNCs such as Merck and GlaxoSmithKline are turned into profitable resources through the direct role of the foundation in disseminating health products sold by these pharmaceuticals in areas such as malaria vaccines, cervical vaccines, and rotavirus and pneumonia vaccines. The role of the foundation in this sense becomes one of creating new markets for TNCs in the health arena by securing access to policy-making structures, state processes, and national-level supply chains without much public accountability because of the tremendous power enjoyed by the foundation simply by virtue of the money being pumped in.

The foundation accomplishes its hegemonic agendas through various forms of partnerships. One key partnership in the vaccine market is with PATH, serving as a space for facilitating the agendas of transnational capital through private partnerships. PATH, funded by the Gates Foundation, collaborates with those transnational private actors through its various projects that the Gates Foundation has significant stakes in. In a document titled "PATH's Guiding Principles for Private Sector Collaboration," the organization notes the following three different pathways of collaboration (PATH, n.d.):

> **Transfer of a technology developed or owned by PATH.** PATH develops a technology in-house and transfers the intellectual property to a private-sector collaborator for further development, manufacturing, and distribution.
>
> **Support by PATH for development of a collaborator's product.** PATH provides significant resources or expertise (such as funding, management, codevelopment, and assistance with clinical studies) to a

> private-sector collaborator to support the collaborator's development of a product.
>
> **Support by PATH for introduction of a collaborator's product.** PATH supports and/or undertakes significant programmatic activities (such as field trials, epidemiological studies, and advocacy programs) that demonstrate and communicate the public health value of a product produced by a private-sector collaborator.

The collaborations of PATH with the private sector are laid out around the agendas of technology transfer to private collaborators and support to private product development through participation in various aspects of product development processes, as well as dissemination support in the form of conducting field trials, epidemiological studies, and advocacy programs. The nonprofit status of PATH under U.S. tax law becomes a facade for carrying out the profit-making agendas of pharmaceutical TNCs. As noted earlier with the role of PATH in promoting the HPV vaccine trials in India, the power structures of PATH and its collaboration with the Gates Foundation, on one hand, and TNCs, on the other hand, create processes of dissemination and operation that are not accountable to state structures, that are not transparent, and that are not shaped by democratic processes of participation. In the case of the HPV trials in India, the economic power of the project obfuscated necessary questions of ethics in the areas of process, transparency, democratic participation, and public accountability.

The power of the Gates Foundation derived through its economic access further works toward pushing specific forms of economic arrangements that benefit the foundation either directly or indirectly. Take, for instance, the large investments of the foundation in Coca-Cola (at the amount of $1.55 billion) and the simultaneous role of the foundation in funding specific forms of local projects in communities in the global South that encourage these communities to become affiliates of Coca-Cola (Stuckler, Basu & McKee, 2011). The partnerships established by the foundation with Coca-Cola raise important questions about the commitment of the foundation to promoting health. The global structures of foundations operate within these very inadequacies, feeding into a global business of technological solutions for health problems that are fostered and reproduced by the very structures of dependence on technologies.

Regulation and Policy Making

The technology fetishism of the foundation simultaneously backgrounds and downplays the role of government policy making and regulations, especially in the backdrop of the large-scale global inequalities that are produced by the neoliberal organizing of global resources, production processes, and economic structures (Millen & Holtz, 2000; Millen, Irwin & Kim, 2000). Whereas the large-scale inequalities, the unequal flow of resources, and the accelerated and massive concentration of power in the hands of the global capitalist elite call for effective national-global regulations, foundations such as the Gates Foundation emphasize modern technologies as solutions to these problems.

Erasures

One of the key arguments put forth by health communication scholars draws attention to the interpretive frames that are circulated in global power structures (Dutta, 2008). When attending to the key frames of global health organizing, not only is it important to critically interrogate the values that are foregrounded and established as normative within these frames, but one must also examine the erasures and absences from the discursive spaces. What has been erased from the discursive space? What is backgrounded? What value frames are missing in the dominant values of market, commodity, and technological fixes offered by technocrats and expert teams that have defined the landscape of neoliberal health governance? In the context of global health, attending to the key global narratives of health circulated by the foundation, attending to the erasures points toward the broader structural contexts within which health is constituted. Absent from the discursive spaces of foundation-speak, for instance, are questions of structural injustice, inequality, and resource redistribution that underlie the large-scale health inequities that have been produced by the very structural adjustments that profit the foundations. For instance, what are the health consequences of sugary-sweet drinks such as Coca-Cola that are promoted toward the youth and children, and especially so in untapped markets in the global South? Interrogating the health effects of Coca-Cola in the contexts of diabetes and obesity, especially in the global South, suggests the contradictory roles of foundations such as the Gates Foundation in creating global markets for unhealthy commodities and at the same time positioning themselves as leaders in the fight for global health.

Clinton Foundation

Another major player in the global health landscape is the Clinton Foundation. The model deployed by the Clinton Foundation is one of social entrepreneurship, offering a complementary model of neoliberal governance that turns social change issues into areas of profiteering, forging markets for facilitation and serving as intermediaries in these negotiation processes. The foundation therefore works to create spaces for business models that take the lessons of the business world to apply to various social change processes. The emphasis on entrepreneurship frames health problems as problems that can be solved through the deployment of management thinking.

Economic Flows

The role of the Clinton Foundation in influencing policies of nation-states across the globe and particularly in the global South is tied to the economic interests that are promoted by the foundation, the economic networks that the foundation is tied to, and to the economic functions served by the foundation. For instance, in 2005, Canadian mining financier Frank Gunstra leveraged the lobbying capacity of Bill Clinton to secure exclusive rights for mining Uranium in Kazakhstan (Youde, 2011). Subsequently, the mining financier donated a total of $131.3 million to the Clinton Foundation (Becker & Van Natta, 2008). Similarly, donors to the Clinton Foundation also served as key fundraisers for Hillary Clinton's 2008 bid for the Democratic presidential elections (Youde, 2011). The flow of capital from powerful actors works to consolidate the role of the foundation as a leverage point for these sources of power. The access to spaces, policy structures, and policy processes across the globe creates economic opportunities for donors into the foundation.

Particularly worth noting are the various conflicts that are generated by the funding flows of the foundation. For instance, one of the funders of the Clinton Foundation is the Coca-Cola Company, donating in the $5 million – $10 million category. Even as the foundation takes money from Coca-Cola, it carries out obesity prevention initiatives under the umbrella of the Clinton Health Matters Initiative. Moreover, the Clinton Health Matters Initiative positions the positive role of corporations as partners in the fight against obesity. This hypocrisy in policy and programming lies at the heart of global neoliberal governance, normalizing the competing logics of the functions and roles carried out by the foundation, its economic structures, and the broader structure of organizing it proposes. The economic ties with transnational corporations that sell health-depleting products (such as Coca-Cola) are whitewashed into health-promoting projects working to find solutions for the very problems that have been created by the sales of these health-depleting products.

Networks of Power

The powerful role played by Bill Clinton as a former president of the United States with strong network ties, along with the role played by his wife, Hillary Clinton, who served as U.S. Secretary of State under Barack Obama, point to the leverage enjoyed by the Clinton Foundation in the landscape of global policy making and programming. These networks of power, building on relationships among global elites, becomes the very point of leverage for the foundation, offering it negotiating powers in crafting out policies and programs on a global scale. As noted by Youde (2011, p. 167), Clinton uses his "personal bully pulpit" to shape global policy agendas. The networks of Clinton with business elites become the basis for the fundamental premise of the foundation in pushing the business model in solving global health problems. The leadership provided by the foundation in bringing private and public leaders together to solve global problems leverages the networks of power, and simultaneously asserts the influence of these networks in directing solutions toward social problems. The power of the foundation lies in turning global social problems created by current power networks into new market opportunities, utilizing terms such as *sustainability*, *win-win relationship*, and *mutual benefits* to create additional domains of privatization (Rauch, 2007).

Promoting the Logic of the Market

At the heart of the work of the Clinton Foundation is its powerful role in pushing the logic of the market as the organizing structure for addressing social change processes. The foundation plays a pivotal role in putting forth ideas of market mechanisms as processes for achieving social change, addressing health issues, and addressing problems of poverty. The ARV price negotiation processes facilitated by the foundation through its Clinton HIV/AIDS Initiative (CHAI), for instance, are celebrated as exemplars of the effectiveness of market-driven mechanisms (Youde, 2011, 2012). CHAI negotiated lower prices of ARVs for a consortium of states, which would directly place their orders with the pharmaceutical manufacturers of generics, thus eliminating intermediaries, ensuring lower prices for states compared with prices in the open markets, and creating larger and stable markets for the generic drugs sold at higher volumes (Shadlen, 2007). The agreements reached by CHAI were with generic pharmaceutical manufacturers in the global South (three in India and one in South Africa), while brand-name TNCs did not show interest in negotiating with the Clinton Foundation (Rauch, 2007). Erased from the articulations of the market are the roles of states, public activism, and global intergovernmental networks in asserting regulatory pressure of pharmaceuticals. The global policy sphere remains unchallenged, keeping intact the profiteering functions of the transnational pharmaceutical industry.

Critical interrogations of the claims made by the Clinton Foundation in bringing down the price of ARVs point out that (a) the foundation ignores the long and arduous activism and confrontational politics by local actors that set the stage for negotiating cheaper ARV prices; (b) there are many organizations that simultaneously worked toward the goal of negotiating cheaper prices; and (c) in the complex scenarios of price mechanisms and negotiations, it is difficult to pinpoint the exact contribution of each of the actors, thus contributing to potential misrepresentation of numbers through double or triple counting (Youde, 2012). The market logic promoted by the foundation suggests solutions in the form of market mechanisms that increase market reach as well as address market inefficiencies through the removal of intermediaries. Erased from the articulations of the market are possibilities of resistance, popular democratic participation, state-driven processes, and global public participatory processes outside the market to drive the prices down. As a result, the foundation not only leaves intact but also promotes the market logic of health, simultaneously undermining the broader structural inequities that constitute poor health.

Similarly, when addressing the issue of climate change, the foundation notes (Clinton Foundation, n.d.), "Together with public and private sector partners, we're proving that measures to fight climate change can also grow economies." The foundation further goes on to note the following:

> Building on President Clinton's longstanding commitment to the environment, the Clinton Climate Initiative (CCI) implements programs that create and advance solutions to the root causes of climate change—while also helping to reduce our reliance on oil, saving money for individuals and governments, creating jobs, and growing economies. CCI, in partnership with the C40 Cities Climate Leadership Group (C40), focuses on helping large cities reduce their carbon emissions. Other programs aim to increase energy efficiency through building retrofits; to increase access to clean energy technology and deploy it at the government, corporate, and homeowner levels; and to reverse deforestation by preserving and regrowing forests.

The topic of climate change becomes a source of profiteering, generating resources, and growing economies. Inherent in the interpretive frames pushed by the foundation is the absence of the articulation of the problematic frames of techno-determinism underlying global problems. Creating jobs and growing economies are tied to reducing reliance on oil and advancing solutions to root causes of climate change. The technology fetish demonstrated by the Gates Foundation is reiterated by the Clinton Foundation in its desire for creating clean energy technology innovations and simultaneously building markets for profiteering for these innovations.

The market logic to social change catalyzed by the Clinton Foundation recirculates the market fundamentalism that dominated the political and economic structures during the Clinton presidency, pushing for structural changes that further consolidated economic power in the hands of transnational capital, weakened unions, weakened government-supported public welfare programs, and further deregulated the U.S. financial economy. It may be argued that the very problems that were produced by the neoliberal reforms carried out by the Clinton administration become the sites of intervention by the Clinton Foundation, ironically offering the same market-driven principles as solutions to these problems in a circuitous logic rife with irony. This depicts the rationality of market fundamentalism where market solutions are recycled as solutions to problems that are generated by the large-scale diffusion of the market logic, thus creating new markets for the commodities and solutions offered within global structures. In critiquing the appearance of Clinton in the 2009 World Economic Forum that addresses global political and economic elites in an invitation to solve the social ills of the world, noted Schwartz:

> I am struck with disbelief with the apparently unlimited extent of their smug arrogance. It is these very men (and yes, they are mostly men!) who are singularly responsible for the mess we are in. [Tony] Blair and Clinton in particular presided over the massive accumulation of debt, reckless deregulation and disproportionate and unbalanced boom in our economy which brought us to the precipice. That they and their ilk imagine that they should now be "sorting things out" is cause for worry. In another time they might have been thrown in the dungeon. It is a powerful statement of our state of affairs that they continue to be so feted. (Schwartz, 2009, quoted in Youde, 2011, p. 174)

Essential to the circulation of the market logic is the powerful role of elite actors in creating innovations that can then be directed at social problems with the goal of addressing them.

Global Health Partnerships

Global health partnerships (GHPs) are organizational structures in the form of alliances, initiatives, and partnerships that bring together private and public actors on a global scale with the goal of addressing health problems (Williams & Rushton, 2011). These partnerships, almost always located in the global North, continue to perpetuate the logics of imperialism that percolated through the development-based framework of global health, locating the centers of knowledge production in the North, developing solutions from the North, and directing these solutions at the global South.

Global health partnerships work hand in hand with foundations; share common objectives, aims, and strategies that are often mutually reinforced through the partnerships; and represent along with foundations a broader global shift in health governance structures toward privatization of solutions, resources, and problems (Williams & Rushton, 2011). The critique of GHPs rearticulates the criticisms of foundations shared earlier, noting that the involvement of the private sector skews the operating framework of the GHPs toward serving private interests. For instance, the Global Fund to Fight AIDS, Tuberculosis, and Malaria, a joint initiative between the G8 and the United Nations secretary-general, formally adopted by the UN General Assembly in 2001, included experts from the pharmaceutical industry on the board of the Global Fund.

The presence of the pharmaceutical industry in decision-making structures of the Global Fund shapes the processes, structures, and outcomes of decisions made in these structures (Rowden, 2009). Noting the intertwined networks of GHPs, WTO, WB, and IMF, who are working in unison to push the global privatization of health, Williams and Rushton (2011, p. 12) share: "All these actors have contributed to significant ideational changes in global health governance—and to a turn in that system towards 'the private'—which have been underpinned by the dominance of neoliberal economics." The claims toward privatization are often based on arguments about (a) filling gaps in global health governance; (b) formation of new sources of expertise and knowledge and; (c) private sector innovations.

Conclusion

Global health foundations have emerged at the center stage of reorganizing global health without a great degree of accountability and transparency built into the structures. The structures of foundations remain opaque with their agendas often tied to the agendas of transnational capitalism. The role of foundations as funding structures for health and health communication projects is critical in the broader context of establishing the culture of self-help, privatization, and individualization of health. Chapter Five will build on the analysis offered in this chapter to specifically examine the role of NGOs.

CHAPTER FOUR

TRANSNATIONAL CAPITAL AND HEALTH

The contemporary frameworks of global organizing of politics and economics shaped by the language of the free market produce a wide variety of detrimental health outcomes. Moreover, global health has increasingly been constituted by the language of the free market, enabled by the powerful role of the state and simultaneously creating corporate structures that now overshadow the power of the state (Millen & Holtz, 2000; Millen, Irwin & Kim, 2000). Governments are key players in pushing the market logic as the framework of organizing health as they seek to attract new opportunities for capital, rationalizing the devolvement of state support for public health programs through the individualization of health risks and the simultaneous creation of new market opportunities in the health sector (Cornia, 2001; Dutta, 2011, 2013a, 2013b). Although paradoxically the free market ideology operates to privatize the public sector through the logic of minimal state intervention, essential to the establishment of neoliberal hegemony is the powerful role of the state in opening up public health resources and infrastructures to the private sector as well as in collaborating with the private sector in many instances to enable its hegemony. The state serves as the harbinger of neoliberalism by implementing a variety of policies, through the use of strategic communication, through the deployment of state power in legislative and executive roles, and through the production of knowledge, as well as through the deployment of violence embodied in state-owned police, paramilitary, and paramilitary apparatuses. Health is framed in terms of individualized risks and privatized responsibility, managed through a variety of private institutions that enable the availability of choices for the activated citizen. These individualized choices make up the demands for privatized products of health that drive the profit structures of TNCs (Labonté & Schrecker, 2007; Labonté et al., 2010; Millen & Holtz, 2000; Millen, Irwin & Kim, 2000; Waitzkin, 1991, 2011).

The large-scale health inequalities that are produced through the implementation of neoliberal policies are managed through the threats of violence often carried out in the hands of the state (Dutta, 2011, 2013a). Resistance to neoliberal policies is either co-opted or controlled with violence through the deployment of partnerships, community engagement programs, police, paramilitary, and the military, as evidenced, for instance, in the large-scale mining operations globally that directly threaten human health. In multiple examples of grassroots resistance to mining operations that have been carried out through the state–private sector nexus, the use of violence has been justified through the framing of resistance as terrorism. States become the primary resource for transnational capital in consolidating power in the hands of capital, and state power provides the legitimacy for the corporatization of resources where the majority of the wealth continues to flow into the hands of the power elite. It is essential to understand the role of communication and information in legitimizing the market through the articulations of the state because ultimately it is through the circulation of specific meanings that the state consolidates power in the hands of transnational capital. Worth interrogating are the linkages between the power elite that continue to flow in and out of corporate structures, structures of governance, and structures of expertise.

In shifting the role of the state in provision of health services, public–private partnerships have emerged as the model for solving health problems under the neoliberal framework of global organizing. In pushing public–private partnerships, international organizations such as the UN as well as national development organizations such as USAID and DfiD have played pivotal roles in funding, implementing, evaluating, and theorizing about the effectiveness of privatization as a model for carrying out global health interventions, often forging entry points for the private sector through partnerships with the public sector. Additionally, a wide array of consulting firms has been deployed to produce knowledge on the potentials of opening up public health infrastructures to the private sector. The production of knowledge has therefore been tied to the implicit agenda of minimizing the role of the state, simultaneously creating new market opportunities for the private sector.

The landscape of global health prevention efforts and health services delivery has been reconstituted under the framework of private–public partnerships, opening up public health to the principles of the market and running public health infrastructures and resources under the principles of markets, management, and privatization. This has resulted in the weakening of public health infrastructures across nation-states even as privatized campaigns driven by the marketing framework have drawn large-scale resources. The privatization of basic health services has rendered these services inaccessible to the poor. Communicating health has been reorganized under the framework of social marketing, shaping health as a commodity to be promoted through branding campaigns, and to be consumed by individual choices. Self-efficacy, defining the belief in the self in the ability to enact individual behaviors, epitomizes the structure of individualized responsibility. Individual-level beliefs and perceived barriers within behavioral contexts are targeted in communication campaigns. Brand associations with private brands, partnerships with commercial products, and product tie-ups are some of the strategies that have been carried out within the organizing principle of privatization.

In this chapter, I interrogate neoliberal policies and programs pushed by the IFIs and WHO, and situate these policies and programs in the backdrop of their effects in the everyday lived experiences of households and communities. I closely interrogate not only the dominant meanings that circulate within these policy and program articulations but also the meanings that are absent from these spaces. I situate the experiences of health constituted by neoliberal policies with the absences in health communication scholarship, thus situating these absences in relationship to the constitutive role of meanings in reproducing the neoliberal order.

Neoliberal Reforms, Governance, and Threats to Health

In this section, I visit the health correlates of neoliberalism in the realm of accelerated consumerism, a marker of globalization processes brought about by neoliberal reforms. I next work through the health literature that documents the health effects of inequalities. Connecting these inequalities with frameworks of global organizing offers an entry point for examining the health consequences of neoliberalism. By fostering a global climate of weak regulatory structures, neoliberalism enables the free flow of health-threatening goods across global borders, powered by the large-scale marketing communication structures deployed by TNCs. The global sale of unhealthy products such as tobacco, sweet drinks, and fast food contributes to the global dominance of obesity, diabetes, and cardiovascular disease. In addition to generating contexts for poor health outcomes, neoliberalism directly impacts health through its relationship to violence. The earliest experiments of neoliberalism carried out in Chile, Nicaragua, and the Philippines were implemented through the violent intervention of the state as an instrument for consolidating power (Harvey, 2001, 2003, 2005). The state worked as a mechanism for achieving the global agenda of transnational capital through funding secured from WB. IMF and WTO played complementary roles in framing the economic structures of the nation-states. Globalization has been coupled with the global dominance of the security and military industries that pose direct threats to human health. The global flow of arms, often carried out ironically in the name of democracy promotion and peace building, directly threatens human health through its relationship with violence.

Neoliberalism and Consumerism

The crisis of neoliberalism, embodied in the U.S. financial crisis of 2008 that catalyzed cascading chains of financial crises across the globe, manifests in the large-scale negative health effects on communities facing the burdens of unemployment, poverty, and food insecurity (Labonté, 2009). One of the key markers of neoliberalism is its model of political economic organizing that privileges massive and accelerated consumption as the framework that drives economic growth. The shortsighted affinities and addictions with consumption are themselves health threats, attached to both adverse physical and mental health outcomes. The ascendance of neoliberalism manifests in accelerated forms of consumption that go alongside with decreasing trust, weakening social affiliations, and weakening networks of belonging (Stiegler, 2010). The short-term consumption affinities of neoliberal societies foster the climate for large-scale and unviable debts, which ultimately result in a variety of other health threats, including the inability to secure access to preventive and primary care, inability to offer educational resources to the next generation, inability to afford health services and health care, and inability to save for long-term health and well-being. The cycles of consumption captured in credit card debts reproduce negative health effects in the forms of stress and various mental health outcomes. Health, treated as a commodity, has to be purchased from the market. Rather than emphasize the forms of basic structures of community health, neoliberal health solutions emphasize technology and innovation that must be continually recycled in transnational networks of production and circulation to generate private profit. Research and development, product design and development, market assessment, and strategic marketing define the ambits of health.

Consumerism emerges as the organizing frame through which health conditions, illnesses, and disease states enter into networks of profiteering. The emergence of direct-to-consumer (DTC) advertising as a communicative device is tied to the neoliberal organizing of health as consumption. Framing the citizen as consumer is intrinsic to the logic of capitalism, and reaching out to a potential consumer segment through segmentation and targeting is the function of advertising. The consumer is made aware of specific health needs that can be fulfilled by the promoted health product. Manufacturing a medical condition through strategic advertising creates the market for the pharmaceutical product. For instance, Pfizer's marketing strategy for selling Viagra works on the underlying cultural fabric, reframing cultural narratives of masculinity and sexuality to construct erectile dysfunction (Baglia, 2005). Narratives of intimacy and relational satisfaction then are reframed by Pfizer in the language of consumption, creating a large market base for Viagra. Communication forms the epicenter of neoliberal marketing of health, shaping needs, desires, and wants that drive the sale of pharmaceutical products.

Responsibility is individualized, with both health communication campaigns and marketing campaigns targeting the individual as a site of intervention (Dutta, 2005). The overarching framework of health communication and the overarching framework of social marketing depict these interpenetrating relationships between individualized responsibility and health outcomes. (In my own early work, depicting my training in the dominant frameworks of social marketing and health communication, I replicate uncritically the notion of individualized responsibility in the form of variables such as health orientation and health efficacy; see Dutta, 2004a, 2004b, 2005.) The individualization of responsibility accomplished through participation in the market is constituted in relationship to a sense of alienation from relationships, from networks of care, from communities, and from collective human responsibilities in networks of affiliation and connection that seek to challenge the individualized greed and selfishness of neoliberal capitalism and foster spaces for alternative forms of imagination guided by commitments to human health and well-being.

Globalization, voiced in the celebratory narratives of the global village, is paradoxically attached to the very forms of atomization, localization, and individuation that narrow down on the individual as the locus of care and control. Participation, defined as essential to health, is branded in walks, marathons, and challenges, detached from the possibilities of participation that organize collectively toward social change (Dutta, 2008; King, 2006). Possibilities of dissent and resistance to the dominant structure are erased as participation gets reframed as consumption. Private philanthropy is mobilized through consumer culture, connecting the responsibility to consume with the responsibility of self-care, positive thinking, and positive connections with other consumers. Relationships fundamentally thus are reframed in the ambits of consumer identities.

Connections with survivors and support networks are constituted in relationship to networks of consumptions, overflowing with brands, slogans, and promotional messages. Responsibility is internalized as self-care, removed from notions of responsibility toward others, toward communities, and toward future generations. Values of selfishness and irresponsible consumption guided by short-term gratification ironically form the communicative features of social marketing campaigns directed at promoting individual responsibility. The rearticulation of irresponsible behavior as individual responsibility is integral to the discursive strategies of neoliberal health communication. Messages of positive lifestyle and self-hope offer the consumerist wish list of new health innovations in the marketplace. Rose (2007, p. 27) notes the following:

> And this moral economy of hope is also an economy in the more traditional sense, for the hope for the innovation that will treat or cure stimulates the circuits of investment. Hence the ethos of hope links together many different actors—or actual or potential sufferers for a cure, of scientists and researchers for a breakthrough that will make their name and advance their career, of doctors and health care professionals for a therapy that will help treat their patients, of biotech companies for a product that will generate profit, of governments for industrial and commercial developments that will generate employment and stimulate economic activity and international competitiveness.

The spaces of "disease communities" and "disease-based support networks" are held together by the capitalist commitments to markets, innovations, and new technologies, all constituted within a broader narrative of profiteering (Rose, 2001, 2007).

Health is paired with a variety of marketing efforts and branding strategies. Disease states form the bases for consumer groups that enter into cycles of advocacy and fundraising, working in partnership with TNCs. Breast cancer, for instance, is strategically framed as a marketing tool in a number of marketing campaigns (King, 2006). The emergence of pink as a brand image is tied to the sales of products ranging from cars to detergents to clothes, framing the moral economy of care as the moral economy of consumption. Notes King (2006, p. 14):

> As the opportunity to participate in raising money for breast cancer research has been used to sell products ranging from Hallmark cards to automobiles, breast cancer marketing has become the focus of much commentary and analysis among marketing experts seeking to understand and chart the passions, interests, and desires of contemporary consumers. Under headlines such as "Cancer Sells," these experts have labeled breast cancer "a dream cause" and pointed to the success of corporate campaigns against the disease as a way to encourage other companies to pursue cause-related marketing.

Cause-related marketing connects the cause to the brand image of the product being marketed, thus creating a positive association with the brand and generating new markets among consumers that are attached to the cause. Marketing efforts targeting "both consumer citizens and corporate citizens" (King, 2006, p. 39) produce citizenship within the ambits of health and intrinsically tied to individualized consumption in the global free market. Buying a brand of automobile or purchasing a brand of yogurt are reframed as acts of participation in the form of volunteerism and charity.

Brand associations create value transference through tie-ups, product placements, event sponsorships, and circulation of logos in marketing campaigns. Consumer products strategically utilize images, such as the pink ribbon, to sell products. Consider similarly the "ice bucket challenge" campaign that went viral on social media, with celebrities such as Bill Gates, Mark Zuckerberg, and George Bush taking up the challenge on social media and pouring a bucket of ice on their heads as a dare directed at generating awareness and funds for research on amyotrophic lateral sclerosis (ALS). The ties of affinity and charitable participation circulated by the challenge obfuscate questions of accountability, expenditure of funds, and the role of the state in supporting research infrastructures. The circuits of participation on social media reify the logics of the dominant structures of neoliberal organizing. Simultaneously erased from discursive spaces are questions of accountability, output, effectiveness, and efficacy, terms that are otherwise central to the efficiency narratives of neoliberalism within the articulations of privatization.

Neoliberalism and Piracy

The logics of privatization in global circuits of capital turn subaltern knowledge into a site of profiteering, simultaneously erasing access in subaltern communities to these forms of knowledge (Dutta, 2011; Shiva, 1988, 1989, 1991; Tsing, 2011). The large-scale production of biological commodities in the free market is married to the institutionalized theft of subaltern knowledge, the removal of such knowledge from the subaltern communities where they originate, the privatization of knowledge claims and the corresponding processes of local knowledge production, and the incorporation of the knowledge claims into global circuits of capitalist production processes as commodities that would extract profit.

The language of innovation is framed within capitalist production as a facade for such forms of biopiracy, leveraging the structure of TRIPS to legitimize and accelerate these global forms of theft as legitimate forms of global business, transnational transactions, and delivery of solutions geared toward delivering health and well-being. Health becomes an instrumental resource of profiteering, tied to biotech incubators, biotech hubs, and bio-incubation experiments. Neoliberal capitalism places emphasis on new innovations and new technologies that would offer new solutions for disease, thus creating new markets for bio-transnationals.

In the desire for profiteering, bio-transnationals deploy a variety of harvesting strategies that capture local knowledge, develop technology-driven innovations derived from such knowledge, and then market these technology-driven products as commodities. As an exemplar of communicative inversion, the very communities that produce subaltern knowledge and have co-constructed this knowledge as a resource for well-being are subject to new logics of exploitation, with their knowledge removed from them and made inaccessible through global market forces. Paradoxically, then, the benefits of local knowledge long circulated within subaltern communities now become out of reach for these very communities, having been introduced into the global circuits of capital and profiteering. The communicative strategies that legitimize theft as innovations driven toward promoting health and well-being are inversions that are structured into knowledge systems, advertising programs, lobbying groups, and a wide variety of public relations strategies.

In another layer of communicative inversion in these processes of biopiracy and resource extraction, the subaltern communities are framed in neoliberal global discourse as primitive and in need of global health interventions, thus offering the framework that legitimizes the expropriation of local knowledge under the language of innovations. Digging deeper into the claims of innovations often renders visible the ties to existing forms of local knowledge that long preceded the biotech experiments. Claims to technology, mass production, and accessibility offer the frameworks of logic that constitute the bulwark of the resource extractive processes in global networks of biopiracy, operating in intertwined networks of institutional structures, state-sponsored laboratories, university research units, private–public partnerships, civil society initiatives, organizations of entrepreneurship, and privatized transnational structures. The role of publicly funded universities is increasingly framed in this space between the public and the private, redefining the role of universities as sites of knowledge production that enable the processes of privatization through their credibility. Simultaneously, knowledge itself becomes an artifact that is privatized and treated as a commodity, with claims of credibility utilized systematically to erase local struggles of resistance, voices of dissent, and alternative arguments that interrogate the value-laden claims of neoliberal structures of knowledge production.

Neoliberal Reforms and Inequalities

The neoliberal restructuring of global economies is organized around the realization and exacerbation of political and economic inequalities, constituted around the hegemonic interpretations of growth-driven development. The metric of growth is seen as the framing device in the ideology of neoliberal economics, circulating the logics of trickle-down economic opportunities that would alleviate poverty. Over the last four decades, neoliberal reforms, carried out across local sites in various forms, have weakened unions and the bargaining power of labor, weakened labor rights, and weakened social welfare programs, which has in turn resulted in large-scale inequalities. These inequalities, primarily measured economically, have also generated enormous health effects, documented in the form of health inequalities within the population as well as low overall population health. Socioeconomic inequalities within communities impact social capital, contributing to low levels of cohesiveness, community participation, and trust, which in turn contributes to poor health outcomes in the community.

A burgeoning body of literature emerges within this context that points to the health inequalities that are witnessed across the globe. Neoliberal health solutions addressing health disparities are framed as solutions of individual choice, targeting individual lifestyles that need to be modified in order to achieve greater health. When the inequalities in health are indeed noted within the neoliberal structures of governance, individual-level behavior modification programs are directed at the targeted communities, often oblivious to the structural contexts of health and the contexts that constitute behavior. Culture is conceptualized as a site of intervention, with effective interventions being conceptualized as culturally sensitive, culturally adapted, and culturally proficient.

Yet another form of neoliberal solutions seeking to address health inequalities emphasizes the role of technologies as solutions to health inequalities. Pointing to the communicative inequalities that mirror health inequalities, these solutions take a techno-deterministic view of communication technologies and networks, privileging communication superhighways as the panacea for health inequalities. Driven by the idea that building the cyberinfrastructure in communities will address health inequalities, these projects fall under the broader framework of digital divide. Absent from a framework of communicative inequality is the structural context of communicative inequality. Thus, within the purviews of neoliberal health communication, inequalities are normalized into the organizing processes of health communication, backgrounding and/or erasing the subaltern claims to knowledge.

Neoliberal Reforms and Unhealthy Products

One of the foundational principles of neoliberalism is the active role of IFIs and powerful nation-states such as the United States and UK in minimizing regulations. Regulations, including health regulations, are framed within neoliberal organizing as threats to free trade, and WTO emerges on the global stage as an adjudicating body. Article XX (b) of GATT that precedes WTO allows member states to take regulatory actions if such actions are necessitated by questions of human life and health. However, as depicted in the case of Thailand's efforts to implement discriminatory taxes on imported cigarettes based on the argument that foreign firms' strong cigarette marketing efforts would overwhelm the public health authorities' antismoking message and thus contribute to the incidence rate of smoking, the GATT panel gave precedence to the free trade logic rather than to the national health needs (GATT, 1991).

The logic of free trade served as the prevailing organizing principle. Moreover, WTO policies put the onus of evidence making regarding health threats on the state, thus reproducing a hegemonic framework that privileges the market over the concerns of health. For instance, the appellate body of WTO ruled that the import ban on beef from hormone-fed cattle violated the WTO agreement governing food and agricultural safety regulations on the basis of objections regarding the lack of appropriate risk assessment (Charnovitz, 2000).

The weakening of national regulations on the flow of unhealthy products and on the advertising and communication of these products targeted at potential audiences has resulted in an environment that enables the global dominance of these unhealthy products, enabled by the organizing principles of the free market. The individualization of responsibility and the framing of lifestyle modification as the site of health communication programs work to shift emphasis away from public accountability and the role of the state in fostering regulatory spaces. Unhealthy products are specifically targeted toward the global South in the search for new markets. In this chapter, we specifically look at the pathways of the global flow of tobacco and unhealthy foods.

Neoliberal Reforms and Displacement

As noted in Chapter Two, one of the fundamental forms of the neoliberal model of profiteering is accumulation by displacement. Large-scale neoliberal reforms have often been carried out through the displacement of subaltern communities from their spaces of livelihood as these spaces have been turned into sites of profiteering. Spaces for industrialization, resource mobilization, and participation have been secured through the displacement of the poor. These displacements have been framed in the language of development, sustainability, bio-conservation, promotion of economic growth, and poverty alleviation. The health effects of displacements are widely documented, resulting in both direct and indirect forms of threat to human health.

Many of the processes of displacement have been realized through local participatory processes, community participatory processes, community workshops, and community engagement programs. The local community emerges as the site of emphasis in the language of participatory communication even as participatory processes are deployed toward serving specific neoliberal agendas framed by WB and IMF. The goals of privatization find new meaning in the ambits of community participatory processes. It is worth noting that the role of participation in neoliberal governance is one of carrying out the agendas of the dominant structures, with community-level engagement activities guided by the impetus to create profits in the market.

Nature and wildlife tourism, offered under a framework of bio-conservation, depict the neoliberalization of nature, wildlife, and agriculture (Münster & Münster, 2012). Therefore, rhetorical frames of land rights and rights to forests have often been deployed precisely as strategies for privatization, positioning private ownership rights toward the goals of privatization of land and natural resources. The language of management of community resources is often played out to co-opt subaltern communities in top-down efforts of privatization of forests, land, and other natural resources (Nayak & Berkes, 2008). Decisions are often already made by policymakers and implementers and then transferred to the communities in the form of joint management. The state, in partnership with the market and civil society, formulates specific management processes that are directed toward co-opting local community participation. Natural resources such as fruits and medicinal plants are introduced into the commodity chain, to be circulated through transactions.

Neoliberal Reforms and Violence

The structural adjustments and political-economic reforms carried out through the pressures exerted by the IFIs are often achieved through the deployment of violence. In the Rwandan genocide in 1994, neoliberal economic reforms played an instrumental role in fostering the bedrock of violence that resulted in large-scale killings (Schoepf, Schoepf & Millen, 2000). Although the meanings attributed to the genocide circulated around age-old colonial frames of tribal conflict that have been narrated through the structures of imperialism, what remains hidden in the broader discursive constructions of the genocide are the underlying economic and political struggles intertwined with struggles for securing control of the state as a resource for enrichment within the broader goals of privatization. The widespread genocide of Tutsi was catalyzed by the racist propaganda by government officials who were being forced to share power amid economic and political struggles resulting from the neoliberal reforms that had ensued in the preceding decade (Schoepf et al., 2000).

On the economic front, in the 1980s, Rwanda experienced WB investments in the form of projects that turned agriculture into an export-driven agricultural economy, often expropriating lands from peasants and privileging large-scale export-driven production on large parastatal tea estates and cattle ranches. On one hand, the projects contributed to a growing crisis in the rural economy by channeling expropriated lands into the hands of elite and bourgeoisie networks; on the other hand, bank expenditures on salary structures, houses for technical advisers, and vehicles further made evident the growing inequality in Rwanda. The money from the development projects went into supporting existing elite structures and further exacerbated the inequalities between the haves and have-nots. Under bank guidelines, agriculture was restructured to export-driven agriculture, with the majority of the resources spent on increasing exports of primarily coffee. The small-scale farms produced insufficient yields and the rural sector experienced land shortage; crop purchasing was left to private merchants and resulted in food price rises.

Poor peasants often fell victim to traders, unable to produce enough food and therefore trading in five bags of coffee worth 30,000 francs in exchange for five bags of beans worth 5,000 francs. The health consequences of poverty and food shortages were evident in the poor health outcomes especially in the rural areas, with high levels of maternal mortality, stunted growth in one-third of the rural children in 1988, and the majority of the health resources spent on training and management efforts. Based on WB recommendations, the "floor price" for coffee paid to coffee growers was withdrawn in 1989, resulting in peasant switches from coffee to food crops and experienced in the form of decline in cash incomes among peasants. In November 1990, Rwanda signed a new SAP agreement with WB, resulting in a 40 percent currency devaluation, accompanied by price increases, debt growth, and decline in production.

On the political front, against the backdrop of the economic struggles, opposition against the single-party government started growing. The government responded to these oppositions through arrests, murders, and harassment. Tutsi refugees, who had fled state-orchestrated pogroms and ethnic cleansing from the 1950s to the 1970s, started crossing the border from Uganda into Rwanda to reclaim their rights under the umbrella of the Rwanda Patriotic Force (RPF). The government responded by arresting approximately ten thousand Tutsi and Hutu political opponents, and by pinning the difficulties on the RPF. As the currency devalued further in 1992, new foreign loans were being deployed toward purchasing weapons and equipment and militarizing the youth. Young men recruited into militias were trained by the army with weapons secured by the government through foreign loans. Hate rhetoric against the Tutsi served as the strategy for the government to consolidate power and to thwart political opposition. What we witness in the Rwandan case study presented here is the large-scale deployment of physical violence that is intertwined with structural violence and the powerful role of the state in constituting neoliberal reforms.

Neoliberalism is accompanied by the growing global investments in the military and in the emergence of the military as an organizing space for health, achieved through the language of geosecurity and global threat. Analyses of the relationship between military spending and mortality suggest that health is negatively related with state allocation of resources to the military. Military spending is negatively correlated with infant mortality rates and life expectancy at birth such that nation-states with greater allocation of resources to the military have higher infant mortality rates and lower life expectancy at birth (Hyatt, 2007). Communication, in the forms of both informational as well as entertainment media, perpetuate the narrative of violence as an organizing frame. Military entertainment, designed in the form of war games and invasions, render commonsensical the neocolonial impetus of global capital.

Neoliberal Reforms and the Private Sector

Neoliberal reforms enable the large-scale transfer of the power of decision making into the hands of the private sector, with minimal regulation exercised by the state. The private sector, as a consequence, consolidates its positions of influence across the globe, simultaneously reproducing and entrenching the communicative and structural inequalities. The neoliberal restructuring of global relations therefore is also a class consolidation, concentrating decision-making structures and processes increasingly into the hands of a small coterie of global elite. That these elites often own resources that cut across finance, media, consumer products, and raw materials speaks to the interconnected networks of power.

Financial Reforms

The neoliberal restructuring of the global political economy is intrinsically tied to the global shifts in power and concentration of capital in the financial sector, with a shift that started in the 1960s and 1970s from the Fordist mode of production predicated on profits as excess of cost proceeds to stock market capitalism that constructed profit as excess of value in the stock exchange (Marazzi, 2010). The state is a key player in the neoliberal restructuring of global political economy, with the U.S. state exerting its imperial role in shaping global financial flows. The United

States worked as a dominant power exerting its influence through Bretton Woods institutions to create the climate for a global free trade system dominated by financial structures (Panitch & Gindin, 2005). The role of the United States at the time of entry into World War II was in fostering global free markets, promoting and fostering free enterprise, and minimizing the barriers to natural expansion. This period saw the hegemonic descent of the U.S. dollar as reserve currency that served as a vehicle through which firms transacted, international exchanges took place, and the value of financial assets was stored. It witnessed the global dissemination of the U.S. financial systems, registering the one-way movement of financial cultures, rules, and rituals, marked by the ascending dominance of fictitious capital (Stiegler, 2010).

A key moment in the financialization of the global economy was the major role played by U.S. investment banks, enabled through the powerful role of the United States, as major spaces for recycling the finances generated from the oil embargo of 1973 and the accompanying OPEC oil price hike (Harvey, 2005). The narrative of development emerged as the catalyst for exerting U.S. imperial influence in opening up new investment opportunities in governments in the global South, framed in the form of development projects (Harvey, 2005; Panitch & Gindin, 2005). Economies in the global South borrowed largely from New York bankers at rates that were established by the bankers, thus leaving the economies vulnerable to rate adjustments imposed by the bankers. Therefore, against the backdrop of U.S. inflation, when the United States introduced the "Volcker shock" in 1979 in the form of rapidly rising interest rates, the Mexican economy went into default in 1982–4. IMF and the U.S. treasury rolled over the debt, manipulating the debt rollover as a strategy for imposing neoliberal reforms in the form of privatization, flexible labor market laws, and cuts in welfare. The structure of neoliberalism revolutionized global financial relationships by placing the ownership of the losses in the hands of the borrower states that were forced by state and global structures to take on board the cost of debt repayment, irrespective of the consequences for the livelihood and well-being of the local population.

Financial innovations, accompanied by innovations in communication technologies, took center stage in the financial reforms of the 1980s. Crises emerged as central to the processes of financialization, with large-scale unemployment that resulted from the crises. As empirically documented through a series of studies on the unemployment generated from the most recent financial crisis, crises have major influences on health, often working through the mediating mechanisms of lack of access to basic health resources, loss of economic capacity to address basic health needs, and the lack of access to health care. The global flows of fictitious capital driven by the twin elements of consumerism and speculation have resulted in the types of effects that fundamentally threaten health and well-being.

Meanings constitute global financialization through the centering of the U.S. currency and the attachment of interpretive frames to U.S. currency, which in turn forms the basis of global transactions. These meanings render as common sense the processes of speculation and fictitious capital, removed from the material bases of production and creation, and rendering as normal the processes of resource extraction that subject savings plans and retirement schemes to networks of speculation, ultimately profiting an elite group of financiers. Speculation as a tool of financial capital thus serves as a tool for resource extraction (primarily salaries put away as monthly savings) from the public.

Employment and Labor

Neoliberal theory operates on the assumption that trade liberalization opens up new opportunities for employment by bringing in new businesses into the country, thus serving as an instrument for poverty alleviation. Yet evidence across countries in the global South documents the loss of livelihoods of millions of workers when the domestic market faces competition from the TNCs with their global reach, globalized production processes, and strong marketing resources. In Chile, net employment fell by 8 percent post-liberalization. Senegal lost one-third of the jobs in the manufacturing sector. Zambia experienced 40 percent reduction in employment in the formal manufacturing sector post-liberalization. Similarly, in the post-liberalization phase in the 1990s, both Malawi and Ghana experienced dramatic falls in employment rates (Christian Aid, 2005; Rowden, 2009). The large-scale job loss in the global South, especially in countries in Africa, relates closely with the rapid deindustrialization of these countries in the face of strong competition faced by the rapid inflow of cheap imports (Rowden, 2009). This rapid deindustrialization is evident in the weakening of the manufacturing sector and the underutilization of industrial capacity, accompanied by unemployment across the globe (United Nations Conference on Trade and Development [UNCTAD], 2006).

Moreover, with trade liberalization, the employment opportunities have mostly shifted to the domain of skilled labor from unskilled labor. With the poor in the global South particularly drawing their livelihoods from the unskilled sector, the rapid liberalization in the South has also meant increasing unemployment among the poorer sections in the global South. The active interventions in government downsizing promoted by IMF have often resulted in large-scale loss of jobs in the formal sector. IMF and WB instructed countries to cut their public sector payroll under the prevailing assumption that the public sectors are inefficient. In many countries across Africa, the introduction of adjustment programs led to the decline in the number of jobs in the formal sector (van der Hoeven, 2000). The loss of jobs from the weakening of the state enterprises actively promoted by the IMF structural adjustment programs did not translate into new economic opportunities for the retrenched workers (van der Geest & van der Hoeven, 1999).

Structural adjustment programs imposed by the IFIs have been instrumental in the weakening of labor rights. The active government downsizing promoted by IMF has dramatically weakened the public sector and fostered large-scale unemployment as the government is the major employer in many countries. Government pension programs across the world have been actively scaled down while at the same time these programs have been privatized through private insurance schemes and privatized social security systems (Rowden, 2009). The privatization of public social security systems has often resulted in less-efficient and less-effective systems as compared with other public systems, with the administrative costs of private systems in Chile and Britain, for example, being 1,500 percent higher compared with the U.S. social security system. The administrative expenses of the privatized system that come in the form of fees and commissions profit the private financial industry and at the same time directly deplete retirement savings of workers.

The "labor flexibility" policies promoted by IMF and WB have translated into the removal of labor protection programs that prohibit employers from firing workers, the removal of minimum wage laws, mandatory wage reduction programs, spreading the gaps between government employees and managers, and the large-scale privatization of pension and social security schemes, with cuts in social security for workers. The notion of labor flexibility operates on the idea that when labor is treated as a commodity, with companies able to hire and fire workers without regulations, markets are able to function efficiently, thus leading to economic growth. The weakening of labor laws and collective bargaining rights place workers in vulnerable situations in global economic flows, with workers having minimal opportunities to have their voices heard, to negotiate minimum wage salaries, and to secure safe working spaces.

Workers as cheap labor have been placed in competition with each other across the globe, with their collective bargaining capacities weakened and/or erased in the name of poverty alleviation and income opportunity. The reproduction of global spaces of production at vulnerable sites across the globe where labor is cheaply available is constituted in the flexibility of movement of production across global boundaries, intensifying work-related health threats globally. Consider, for instance, the large number of worker deaths at the garment factory in the Rana Plaza in the Savar district of Bangladesh, produced as a result of unsafe building structures in an unregulated environment (*Guardian*, April 23, 2014). The garment industry, a major employer in Bangladesh, operates in global circuits of profiteering, with extremely low wages that are unregulated, poor construction standards, and hazardous working environments, and it depicts the health threats that are posed by neoliberal flows of global capital, production systems, and manufacturing processes. Similarly, the deaths of workers at construction sites across the globe point toward the poor regulatory standards alongside salient threats to worker health in high speed processes of construction (Booth, 2013). In addition to being exposed to workplace hazards and unsafe working environments, workers often have no or limited access to health insurance, treatments for work-related injuries, or compensations for injuries related to work (Heinsman, 2011). Across the global margins from the North to the South, workers in the informal sector often are not covered by health insurance (Heinsman, 2011).

Questions of labor, worker rights, rights to health and health care, collective bargaining rights, and rights to minimum wage remain absent from the discursive spaces of neoliberal globalization and from the meaning frameworks of the dominant health communication scholarship, even as the rights discourse percolates across the structures of neoliberalism. With the weakening of public health infrastructures across global spaces directed by IFI-led initiatives of reforming the health sector, the accompanying weakening of worker rights renders workers vulnerable at multiple levels. Health communication as an organizing structure of interpretations is silent about the organizing of labor in the context of structural reforms imposed by the IFIs, instead focusing on work-life balance, self-help programs, and workplace-based individually directed lifestyle interventions. Behavior modifications such as stress reduction through meditation and self-awareness reify the neoliberal emphasis on the individual in the workplace, simultaneously erasing questions of collective bargaining.

Extractive Industries and the Nation–State

Neoliberal capitalism has facilitated the growth of global network flows that extract mineral resources from distant spaces in the global South to be incorporated into the global flows of capital. Neoliberal reforms were central to the organizing role of WB in shaping the economic policies of African nation-states. One of the ways in which SAPs imposed their economic reforms on African states was to impose specific procedures and processes of mineral resource extraction, enabling the extractive roles of TNCs. Governments were pushed by WB to grow the extractive industries, often without consultation with local people and local communities, and often at the cost of tremendous health threats to local communities. The power of the extractive industries is often exerted through collaborations with teams of experts, civil society organizations, and state authorities that work together to frame the knowledge claims at sites of contestation. Claims to economic development and employment are often juxtaposed against questions of health, carried out with a variety of communication tools, such as reports and studies, that offer the facade of objective knowledge. As forms of communicative inversion, such frames of knowledge claims often pick particular elements to render salient while at the same time erasing other elements.

The environmental effects of drilling and mining operations include air and water pollution, in many instances leading to adverse health effects (the wide array of environmental effects is discussed in the next section). Even as local community health suffered as a result of the very functions of extraction, TNCs partnered with local NGOs and community organizations to deliver health solutions, health tests, and educational programs. As an exemplar of communicative inversion, positive contribution to local health through community consultation, engagement, dialogue, and participation is juxtaposed against the backdrop of the large effects on health caused by the extractive industries (Farsetta, 2010).

Local communities experiencing the negative effects of the extractive industries voice the everyday health experiences reproduced on the cartography of the body. As protests started growing across nation-states in the African continent, governments increasingly responded through the deployment of violence, incorporating state-funded and private military to thwart dissent. The poverty-producing effects of the SAPs were integral to the protests against price rise and unemployment across various states in Africa. Clubbed under the term *IMF riots*, the protests were dealt with through the use of force (this is discussed in greater depth in Chapter Six). The strong presence of the military in Nigeria and the deployment of violence to control dissent is a key theme in the context of Shell's operations in Ogoniland in Nigeria. As local communities started to protest the health and environmental effects of the drilling operations, the state carried out systematic violence to enable the continued operation of Shell. Shell subsequently participated in a variety of public relations activities framed as "sustainable development" to clean up its image.

Global Warming, Pollution, and Threats to Health

Human causes of global warming and climate change have generated health burdens that are unequally borne across the international lines of division of labor, with the global South bearing major burdens in the form of floods and extreme weather events, manifesting in direct threats to human health and well-being. The burdens of these weather events are mostly borne by the poor, with associated health impacts that are disproportionately felt by the poor. Polluting industries such as the oil and fossil fuel industries leave major impacts on the environment, contributing to global warming, affecting water quality, and severely impacting air quality.

Neoliberal interventions emphasizing profiteering and free flow of capital often undermine the health and environmental impacts of transnational corporations. Knowledge is framed within industry agendas, with academics often working on the payroll of TNCs. For instance, within the context of climate change, funded by the fossil fuel industry, and operating within the nexus of foundations and think tanks, experts with scientific credentials are engaged to "keep the controversy alive" (Oreskes & Conway, 2010, p. 5). Keeping the controversy alive works as a barrier to regulation of the fossil fuel industry. Even as science uses the language of value-free science free from politics, the institutions and structures of science are constituted in these networks and relationships of power that are married to specific policy outcomes.

The case of global warming depicts the ways in which oil corporations and the broader fossil fuel industry carry out a variety of public relations tactics, including hiring academic experts, funding university research, hiring lobbying groups, attaching with NGOs that facilitate the efforts of green washing, and working with political leaders to circulate misleading information on global warming. Expertise plays a fundamental role in shaping the realms of knowledge claims, with networks of experts funded by the industry. Questions of conflict of interest, flows of power in processes of publishing, and the biases that are introduced into science through the mechanisms of funding are systematically erased. Communication works to render as normative issues of industry funding, often on the basis of the argument that funding is needed to carry out studies.

Privatization of Water and Natural Resources

As transnational capital scans and seeks new market opportunities in the form of entrepreneurship and private–public partnerships, natural resources such as water and air emerge as sites of corporate control and profiteering. Large TNCs such as Coca-Cola and Pepsi operate in globally distributed local spaces of production, often needing large supplies of water to feed the production processes. Communities in the global South experience shortage in water supplies as water tables are depleted by corporate manufacturing plants. Paradoxically, TNCs deploy communicative inversions through CSR programs, sustainable development projects, and community-grounded participatory collaborations in conjunction with civil society organizations that are framed as projects of building water capacities. The transnational hegemonic control on water supplies was evident in the privatizing initiatives carried out by Bechtel in Cochabamba that was directed at privatizing the water resources. Nestle invests heavily into the privatization of water, also working toward shaping the global policy environment. The privatization of water fundamentally threatens health by introducing water into the networks of capitalist flow and by removing access to water from underserved communities. Neoliberal health interventions often strategically reproduce the narrative of increasing community access to natural resources such as water and air to justify processes of commoditization and privatization.

Privatization of Agriculture and Threats to Health

One of the major areas of neoliberal intervention has been the commercialization of agriculture, transforming agriculture from food-driven forms of local, culturally rooted, sustainable organizing to cash-driven forms of organizing, captured in the hands of global agrochemical transnationals such as Monsanto and delivered in the form of development interventions (Clapp, 2012). The promise to feed the world's poor has offered the facade for corporatization of agriculture, consolidating the agriculture sector in the hands of agro-TNCs. Structural adjustment programs imposed by WB and IMF have imposed harmonization plans that have opened up the agricultural sector to transnational corporations, often erasing local small-scale farmers and farmworkers from spaces of participation in local agriculture. Notes Clapp (2012, p. 22):

> The world food economy has been shaped by key forces that have, as the world food system has become more globalized, managed to create and occupy middle spaces in that system. The opening up of these spaces by governments, private foundations, TNCs, and financial actors has created new norms and governance frameworks, including international trade rules that have shifted control away from farmers and consumers and toward the center. As this process has occurred, new features of the world food economy has emerged, including the commodification of food and the problem of distance, imbalance and volatility in world food markets, and ecological crisis linked to the industrialization of agriculture that serves the global system.

Communication as the circulation of meaning lies at the heart of these global processes of diffusion of agriculture biotechnologies (Brossard,

Shanahan & Nesbitt, 2007). Local forms of knowing are constructed discursively as primitive and therefore in need for modernization, understood in the form of agricultural innovations such as new seed technologies, irrigation technologies, farming technologies, pesticides, fertilizers, and so on. The innovation thus comes from the commercialized center of knowledge production, disseminated as a solution that needs to be purchased by farming communities at a steep price.

Biotechnology is one such innovation that is offered to the global South as a solution to problems of food insecurity and hunger. As the development model of biotechnology dissemination has transformed into the neoliberal model of dissemination, development actors such as USAID operate within a collaborative framework with agro-transnationals such as Monsanto, public and private research institutions such as universities, and a wide array of NGOs. The public–private partnerships that are often directed at delivering biotechnology solutions carry out the agendas of privatization under the facade of public and civil society collaborations. The knowledge of the expert, framed as a modernizing tool, is juxtaposed with the primitive knowledge of the recipient communities, constructing the modern–primitive dichotomy in a racist frame. The array of experts that are deployed to carry out the interventions are often paid for by private capital, thus constituting the processes of knowledge production within the structures and agendas of transnational capitalism.

Fast Food Industry, Food and Beverage Transnationals, and Health

The opening up of economics across the globe has been accompanied by the rapid global movement of unhealthy foods marketed by TNCs located in the West, pushed through the free market framework promoted by IFIs. The global penetration of fast food is attached to the search for new markets for TNCs operating in the fast-food sector, leveraging an array of marketing and public relations strategies (Nestle, 2013). The role of communication is integral to the marketing functions of advertising agencies and public relations transnationals that fine-tune persuasive strategies to target potential audiences across the globe, creating new global markets for a variety of fast-food products, developing the right mix of local adaptation and global standardization that delivers the brand appeal.

The volume of global food advertising expenditure speaks to the communicative power exercised by food transnationals. Hawkes, Chopra, and Friel (2009) reported the more than doubling of global food advertising expenditures from US$216 billion in 1980 to US$512 billion in 2004 (World Watch, cited in Hawkes et al., 2009, p. 253). Food advertising globally constitutes one of the largest sectors of advertising, with increasing budgets of food advertising directed toward developing countries. Growing "new" markets form the bulwark of FTCs, such as the Coca-Cola Company, considered as one of the top ten largest spenders in developing countries. Advertising for poor-quality, high-calorie, nutrient-poor processed foods takes up most of the advertising space, directed toward children, and often in the form of television advertising.

The four Ps of marketing—product, price, promotion, and place—drive strategies that seek to create new needs, desires, and affinities targeting countries in the global South, and often with an emphasis on children and youth. Neoliberalism fosters a privatized model that brings in transnational capital in partnership with spaces such as schools where children are exposed to products such as soft drinks early on, creating spaces of brand loyalty and brand affinity in the formative years of life. Much of the food advertising and promotion is targeted at children and youth, often selling high-calorie, nutrient-poor foods (Hastings et al., 2006; Stead et al., 2003). A key element of the marketing model is "place," and the food industry secures a captive place for the marketing of food products in schools, incorporating strategic "partnerships" as key elements of the marketing mix, especially within the context of new and emerging markets. As transnational corporations have secured entry into schools, education has been incorporated into the branding logics of food-based TNCs, with vending machines and food programs serving as sites of delivery of food products. Neoliberalism in a nutshell has served as the primary player in the unregulated global circulation of unhealthy foods and large amounts of advertising/communication/marketing expenditures on pushing these unhealthy foods.

Tobacco and Liberalization

With the liberalization of global trade, the free flow of tobacco across global borders has brought about disproportionate health risks in the global South, with smoking incidence increasing dramatically in lower-income countries (Yach et al., 2008). Tobacco-related health diseases are predicted to kill more than ten million people every year by 2030, with 70 percent of these deaths taking place in middle- and low-income countries (Yach et al., 2008). The big advertising budgets of the tobacco industry accompanied by the influences of global branding popularized the image of the Marlboro man as a global signifier of desire. Add to that the advertising dollars that drive communication campaigns promoting tobacco and the public relations efforts of large TNCs in recruiting experts in shaping knowledge claims and in driving large-scale lobbying efforts that seek to buy off political leaders typically in the form of campaign financing.

The influence of the global tobacco industry in the form of aggressive lobbying shapes the regulatory environment around tobacco, resulting in a lack of adequate regulatory mechanisms for controlling the sale of tobacco in spite of the direct effects on heath. Even as governments in the power centers in the global North have introduced anti-tobacco campaigns, public service announcements, and special policies to regulate the tobacco industry, nation-states in the global South increasingly emerge as targets of tobacco marketing. Unequal access to the influence structures of IMF, WB, and WTO are mobilized by the transnational tobacco corporations (TTCs) to open up markets for tobacco.

The global expansion of the harmful health effects of privatization is well evident in the context of tobacco, with the free market logic offering the legal, political, and economic pathway for the global flow of tobacco trade, and simultaneously erasing opportunities for health regulations grounded in articulations of human health. Liberalization has resulted in the powerful influence of the IFIs in opening up open trade areas in Asia and Latin America (Hammond, 1998). In addition, the structures of IFIs, mainly WB and IMF, have been leveraged by powerful TTCs to exert pressure on countries to privatize state-owned tobacco companies and to liberalize foreign investment laws. Moreover, in one of the most poignant accounts of the harmful health effects of neoliberal globalization, the opening up of closed economies such as the Soviet Union, Eastern Europe, and China have resulted in pressure exerted by IFIs to privatize their state-owned industries and liberalize their economies, which in turn resulted in large-scale investments by TTCs in new and emerging local markets across the globe.

Communication has played a key role in the processes of global expansion of TTCs. Rebranding strategies and corporate social responsibility programs have worked toward cleaning up the images of TTCs. In exemplars of communicative inversion, TTCs have worked with communication management corporations in shifting their image toward health. For instance, associations with health causes have created new market opportunities for TTCs. The media–tobacco industry linkage offers another powerful example of the poor health effects of transnational hegemony caused by the collaborations between transnational corporations and transnational media organizations. Phillip Morris has long enjoyed a strong relationship with Rupert Murdoch (see Burton, 2007).

Militarization and Threats to Health

Wars and violence carried out by the military constitute fundamental forms of threat to human health (Levy & Sidel, 1997). The militarization of the globe under the framework of fighting terrorism is intrinsic to the neoliberal apparatus, strengthening the military apparatus that maintains the power and control of the global elite (Waitzkin, 2011). The power of the state as an instrument of control is further reified in the global role of the state as a site of imperial power, working to protect the interests of TNCs globally. The logics of war are often constituted within imperial agendas of securing power and control over oil and other forms of natural resources (Harvey, 2003).

As evidenced in the examples of Iraq and Afghanistan, the U.S. state emerges as a power that exerts its control through the military, and it does so within a broader logic of economic opening up. The human rights abuses witnessed in Operation Iraqi Freedom and in the war in Afghanistan document the threats to human health that are posed by militarization. Military violence creates markets around the globe for military commodities manufactured by military TNCs (MTNCs) operating in the arms and weapons sectors. Wars and efforts of fighting terror thus feed the markets of arms-based TNCs. Similarly, infrastructure-driven TNCs find new market opportunities in war-ravaged zones where large grants become available for carrying out the tasks of reconstruction.

The neoliberal narrative of governance works through the framing of terrorism as a risk to the nation-state, simultaneously working to consolidate tremendous levels of control in the hands of the military by perpetuating the narrative of geosecurity. Military interventions fundamentally threaten human health, directly impacting both mortality and morbidity. Forms of violence in the form of imprisonment and torture are sites of power and control within the military-industrial complex. The privatization of the military in the arena of geosecurity provides new business opportunities for private actors in the security arena. The media work hand in hand with transnational capitalism and with the military to frame agendas for military intervention, circulating specific frames that support military interventions and simultaneously erasing or backgrounding critical questions. Communication is continually at work to justify these military interventions, recycling the propaganda of dominant political, economic, and social actors, and simultaneously generating new business opportunities for MTNCs. Entertainment programming and persuasive messaging on digital media serve as military engagement strategies.

Pharmaceutical Industry and Neoliberalism

The global shifts in health organizing based on neoliberal values is witnessed in the ascendance of the pharmaceutical industry as a powerful global force, mediatized through the dominant role of the market, enabled by the active role of the nation-state in securing markets for pharmaceutical TNCs.

Pharmaceuticals, with their large-scale marketing, advertising, public relations, and advocacy strategies, play pivotal roles in creating ontological categories of disease, in marking these categories as sites of clinical research and interventions, and in marketing products directed at addressing these needs. The individual consumer as a rational decision-making agent is the unit of decision making, and is bombarded with plethora of advertising promoting various brands of pharmaceutical solutions, complemented by marketing regimens directed at providers. The pharmaceutical market, increasingly removed from evidence-based science, is captured through well-packaged marketing campaigns that present unique selling propositions to the consumer.

New disease formations such as social anxiety disorder, panic disorder, and attention deficit disorder are presented and marketed widely, and miracle pharmaceutical solutions to these disorders are positioned through advertising. Individual consumers are encouraged to participate, to ask their doctors to prescribe the medication, and to solve their newly identified health problems through the consumption of the health products. Health providers in turn are actively targeted as agents for pushing the pharmaceutical products, enticed through gifts, sponsored trips, and specialized packages. The scientists who carry out the research and publish the results of clinical trials are often themselves incorporated into the logics of the market, funded by the pharmaceuticals. The incorporation of clinical trials and ghostwriting into the marketing logics of the pharmaceutical industry depict the neoliberal restructuring of health (Healy, 2007). Data on adverse effects, such as suicidal attempts and completed suicides, for instance, are omitted from the published academic research.

The TRIPS under WTO protect patents across national borders, mandating that all WTO countries implement intellectual property protections, providing owners and developers a twenty-year monopoly over patentable products. Working through the powerful instruments of the state, pharmaceutical TNCs maneuver the TRIPS to safeguard their products in global markets, thus maintaining monopoly over the market for a sustained period of time where the profits flow to the pharmaceutical TNCs. Publicly funded programs such as U.S. Medicare and Medicaid had to pay substantially higher prices because of the twenty-year patent policy. Waitzkin (2011) argued that TRIPS substantially impacted U.S. health care cost containment measures by extending the time period for which users had to pay high prices for patented medications.

In the context of global flows of medicines, intellectual property rights are deployed to constrain the manufacturing of generics in the global South at cheaper prices, framed within the narrative of protecting and enabling innovations. The patenting laws of TRIPS place limits on the extent to which generic versions can be developed and circulated in the global South at prices that are accessible to the poor and lower-middle-class families for whom basic medicine is already an expensive commodity. In a study of the generic market of quinolones in India, Chaudhuri, Goldberg, and Panle (2003) estimated annual welfare losses of $305 million that would result if quinolones, a subsegment of the antibacterial segment of the Indian pharmaceutical market, were under patent in India as they were in the United States, while the profits under the existing price regulations to the foreign producer would have been around $19.6 million per year. Similarly, other scholars noted the much higher prices that patients would have to pay in developing countries with the introduction of patent laws, thus limiting access to medicine among the poor and reducing welfare in developing countries (Scherer, 2004).

The "compulsory licensing" policy under TRIPS offers nation-states the flexibility of allowing third-party manufacturers to produce the patented product or process without the consent of the patent owner, although a fee will have to be paid to the patent owner. The United States, serving as an instrument for U.S.-based pharmaceutical TNCs, supported efforts under TRIPS to prevent Indian, Brazil, Thailand, and South Africa from initiating compulsory licenses for production of generic versions of AIDS medications under patents. Depicting the inherent contradictions of neoliberal policies, even as the United States aggressively resisted "compulsory licensing" arrangements in the global South, it domestically applied a number of "compulsory licensing" arrangements locally in response to anticompetitive practices.

The irony in the neoliberal structuring of global health problems lies in the powerful role of the state in allocating public resources (paid in the form of taxes) to fund research that is then turned into private commodities for pharmaceutical profits. Neoliberal organizing of pharmaceuticals replicates the broader structures and processes of neoliberalism that designate the state as the protector of commercial interests in the name of the market, as well as an enabler for channeling public resources paid in the form of taxes to serve private interests, framed in the form of research and development. In this sense, the state is an active player in the rent-extracting processes, channeling public resources into the market, which then sells the commodities developed from these very resources to the public at a profit. The profit extracted by TNCs is derived from large shares of public resources that are allocated for purposes of business development by the state.

In his analysis of the postindustrial proliferation of the biotechnology industry in nodal centers such as Hyderabad in India, Sunder Rajan (2006) draws our attention to the role of the Chandrababu Naidu government of Andhra Pradesh to simultaneously use the language of political and economic decentralization to promote a biotech hub, the ICICI Knowledge Park, in an area designated by the government as the "Genome Valley" for the promotion of biotech innovation. The Park, replete with biotechnology infrastructure, is a collaboration between the Andhra Pradesh government and the venture capital and financial services company ICICI, with the goal of serving as a source of high quality scientific labor for multinationals interested in doing research in India. Sunder Rajan notes the contradictions between the rhetoric of promoting biotechnology innovation that serves as the discursive legitimation for the Park and the practice of extracting cheap biotechnology labor utilizing state-subsidized infrastructure to serve the commercial interests of biotechnology capital located in the West.

Privatization of Health

In this section, we attend to the adjustment policies promoted by IMF, WB, and WHO in the arena of health. The neoliberal reforms of the health sector have specifically focused on reconstituting the health sector in the logics of privatization. State-supported public health systems have been specifically targeted under programs of privatization, creating new markets for the insurance industry and the managed care sector. Essential to the organizing logic of privatization is the framing of privatizing processes as solutions to problems of global health. The framing of the public sector as inefficient and incapable and the devaluation of public sector programs are intrinsic to the processes of privatization through public–private partnerships (PPP).

Public–private partnerships (PPPs) in health have become the dominant framework of health organizing within the constitutive structure of neoliberalism. WHO, as a key actor in the development of the global health agenda, frames health in terms of the role of private corporations in managing privatized risks, and simultaneously shifts the onus of accountability into the hands of private corporations. Consider, for instance, the following from a position paper on PPPs (Buse & Waxman, 2001, p. 749):

> WHO is inevitably engaged in various types of interaction with the private sector, many of them desirable and necessary. The tobacco industry, for example, participated in public hearings organized by WHO in October 2000 on the Framework Convention on Tobacco Control and its experts contribute regularly to the WHO Scientific Advisory Committee on Tobacco Product Regulation. WHO's interactions with the private sector range from working with employees of companies who act in their personal expert capacities or are seconded from companies to participate in decision-making bodies, to engaging

> in more formal partnership arrangements (i.e., based on bilateral legal agreements).

Worth observing here is the role of WHO in shifting the point of accountability into the hands of private corporations such as the tobacco industry, the very industry that is being targeted for regulation because of its health-threatening impacts (Marmot & Wilkinson, 2006).

In spite of the large body of evidence that documents the role of the tobacco industry in fighting regulations seeking to hold the tobacco industry accountable, the participation of the tobacco industry as a partner in the regulatory process turns the process into a collaborative instrument that works in tandem with the agendas of the industry. The very meaning of *regulation* is rendered meaningless by the participation of the targeted industry in the regulatory processes. The role of tobacco industry experts as contributors to the Framework Convention on Tobacco Control works paradoxically to regulate the agendas of the industry through the very participation of the industry, thus ultimately serving the agendas of the industry. The framing of expert knowledge in the hands of private industry experts further turns WHO knowledge within the ambits of the private sector, constituting the parameters of health governance within the domains of privatized expert knowledge.

Another such irony in the WHO position is depicted in the predominant role of the private industry as a solution presented in the WHO report on social determinants of health titled *Closing the Gap in a Generation*. The report eloquently points toward a number of structural features of the environment that constitute health and yet shies away from putting forth among its recommendations for addressing the structural determinants of health a framework for regulating the financialization of health, the health-threatening industries, and the global flows of unhealthy commodities. Instead, proposing the private sector as part of the solution, it goes on to outline the following: "Reaching beyond the government to involve civil society and the voluntary and private sectors is a vital step towards action for health equity. The increased incorporation of community engagement and social participation in policy processes helps to ensure fair decision-making on health equity issues" (WHO, 2008, p. 10). Note here the incorporation of community participatory processes and community engagement within the dominant structures of private, civil society, and public alignments. Absent from this discursive space are articulations of local community participatory processes in antagonistic or confrontational relationships, holding accountable the structures of civil society and the private sector. The framing of the relationship among the state, civil society, and private sector in a partnership relationship is one of the fundamental health-threatening effects of neoliberal governmentality, weakening the structures of debate, confrontation, and accountability in the relationships among these key elements of governmentality.

Social marketing as a health solution organizes the dominant framework of health communication in a global scale, organizing discourse and meaning in the language of the consumer, wants, brand positioning, and message appeal. Communicating about health is conceived as an analogy between the private sector and the public constructions of health-based social change, privileging the logic of the market, constructing the individual as a health consumer, putting forth a managerial model, and targeting the health consumer through the strategic deployment of the marketing mix. Promotion, working in tandem with product, place, and price, offers the guiding framework for addressing individual-based (un)healthy lifestyles that are targets of social marketing campaigns. Eating fruits and vegetables, exercising, and tobacco cessation are seen through this lens of lifestyle modification, framing the discussion in the language of health communication strategy constituted in the marketing mix. Simultaneously, discussions of unhealthy structures, the structural elements that organize health and health care, and the capitalist logic that is intertwined with the organizing principles of the structures are absent from the discursive space. The private sector emerges as a partner through co-branding and message alignment strategies, thus capturing health in a close relationship with the market. Reifying the communicative inequality that constitutes neoliberal organizing, expert-driven messaging strategies are designed to serve the goal of effective behavior change.

The hegemony of the neoliberal logic narrows down on the individual, localizing the problem to a targeted lifestyle, belief, attitude, or behavior. Such aggressive targeting and narrow focus on the individual obfuscates the interconnected networks of power that constitute health. As has been articulated throughout the various sections of this chapter, the logics of individualization and privatization work well when they specifically target single issues and frame these issues in terms of technological innovations that would solve them, thus reiterating the technology fetish of neoliberalism. Resisting this narrowly individualistic framework of neoliberal health organizing calls for close interrogation of the taken-for-granted assumptions of health and communication about health.

Conclusion

This chapter offers a close reading of the interpretations, frames, meanings, and discourses that are constituted within global structures of neoliberalism.

The narratives of individualism, self-care, and commoditization that run through transnational structures of neoliberal organizing depict the collaborative relationships among the transnational elite as well as the powerful role of the state as the key actor in carrying out neoliberal reforms. The communicative inequalities and inversions in neoliberal discourse depict the role of strategic communication in reorganizing global relationships, simultaneously minimizing the opportunities for participation among the subaltern sectors of the globe. The ecology of global health is fundamentally threatened through neoliberal reforms that impact every aspect of human life ranging from access to agriculture and food, access to natural resources, right to a clean and sustainable environment, right to education, right to work and employment opportunities, and right to fundamental health care. Closely considering the health effects of neoliberal governance point toward the adverse health effects of industries such as tobacco and fast-food industries, adverse health effects of consumerism, adverse health effects of financial reforms, and the fundamentally health-impeding effects of police and military violence deployed toward serving neoliberal hegemony.

CHAPTER FIVE

NGOS, HEALTH COMMUNICATION, AND DEMOCRACY

The organizing of health within neoliberalism has worked specifically through the articulation of the state, civil society, and market linkage as essential to the formulation of health policies and health practices. Meanings of health have been framed in the logic of the market, with civil society operating as a primary actor working in partnerships with the market in delivering essential health services, in diverting resources away from public health programs, and in privatizing them through models of empowerment (Petras, 1999). Essential to the global hegemony of neoliberalism was the acknowledgment of global poverty as a problem and the simultaneous conceptualization of the role of civil society in addressing poverty (Ibrahim & Hulme, 2011).

Health of the poor emerged as a site for privatized interventions. As core players in civil society, NGOs have played vital roles in the privatization of health, emerging on the landscape as the key resources for delivering health, simultaneously minimizing the role of the state as the point of delivery of public health and public health care (Kamat, 2004; Pfeiffer & Chapman, 2010). NGOs funded by global imperial structures have been instrumental to the circulation of the logic of neoliberalism, threatening the welfare functions of the state and simultaneously creating new markets in the arena of social services through logics of self-help and empowerment (Petras, 1997, 1999). The weakening of the state and state services is integral to the strengthening of the NGO sector amid large-scale neoliberal reforms, with the NGO sector taking on the role of delivering services for the poor in the absence of public structures, welfare, and public health capacities.

The consistent decrease in the expenditure of public resources in providing for basic capabilities of health has been married to the emergence of private–public linkages that have taken center stage in the delivery of health services (Doyle & Patel, 2008). Therefore, the appearance of NGOs on the global political landscape is intrinsically tied to the declining role of the state as a provider of social welfare and public health services (Kaldor, 2003; Powell, 2007). Interrogating the active role of NGOs in the consolidation of power in the hands of transnational capital, Kaldor (2003, p. 88) observes:

> Markets plus elections became the ideological formula of the 1990s. NGOs came to be seen as an important mechanism for implementing this agenda. They can provide a social safety net without extending the role of the government.

NGOs, with their funding structures intrinsically tied to the international funding structures located in the global North, have carried out the agendas of these funding structures in liberalizing markets, minimizing state subsidies, de-unionizing workers, and weakening the state-driven sectors (Kaldor, 2003; Powell, 2007). Health has emerged in this NGO discourse in the language of privatized entrepreneurship, with emphasis on terms such as *empowerment*, *self-efficacy*, *community empowerment*, and *individual participation* (Kamat, 2004; Pfeiffer & Chapman, 2010). The localization of health has been achieved through the ownership of responsibility at the level of the community with community-driven projects taking up the language of empowerment to deploy funds, top-down agendas, and implementation processes. Terms that appear to be emancipatory, such as *community participation* and *community engagement*, have emerged as tropes for carrying out the liberalization of health, with the devolvement of state-based infrastructures in the provision of basic health and health care. NGOs emerge as elite-driven structures for carrying out the agendas of transnational capital at the grassroots, simultaneously erasing the possibilities of popular participation, resistance, and structural transformation of the broader organizing processes of neoliberalism, neutralizing the transformative potential of popular politics (Kaldor, 2003).

It is particularly salient to look closely at the communicative processes that are carried out in the NGO-driven discourse (London & Schneider, 2012). The community emerges as the site of the intervention and community participatory processes are incorporated into structures of decision making, suggesting a grassroots-driven and bottom-up alternative to top-down expertise-based decision structure (Wilson, Lavis & Guta, 2012). Organizational forms such as community-based organizations emerge as structures for the delivery of health at the community level, serving as interfaces with community structures and participatory processes. The NGO emerges in global health structures of neoliberal governance as the face of the community, developing a variety of community-based participatory processes that are driven by the funding agendas of donors. The nature and texture of participation in these NGO processes is constituted within the top-down frameworks and goals of funding agencies. The community becomes a conduit for carrying out privatized health solutions achieved through the participation of the individual consumer into the market. The emergence of the NGO sector as a site for the delivery of health has also simultaneously fostered global spaces for human rights discourses, offering entry points for the articulation of health as human rights. As we argue in the concluding section of this chapter, whereas the human rights framework has been integral to the privatization of health, it has also fostered openings for advocacy and activism in the realms of arguments of rights to preventive services, health resources, health services, and health care.

The individualization of health problems evident in early modernization discourses of development reflecting the capitalist roots of development politics are further entrenched into the structures of public–private partnerships, and NGOs are pivotal in carrying out these partnerships locally. The global framework of solutions to health problems frames health in the realm of individual beliefs, attitudes, and behaviors, and simultaneously erases underlying questions of resource distribution, lack of access to basic resources, and the large-scale inequalities that are generated by growth-driven globalization processes. NGOs therefore are a key element of the neoliberalization process, being integral to the minimized role of the state in delivering health services and simultaneously placing the emphasis on the individual and his or her behaviors as solutions to health problems.

In sum, NGOs have emerged on the landscape of neoliberalism as spaces of organizing resources, as structures for enabling private–public linkages, and as outlets for carrying out the broader agendas of privatization of health (Kamat, 2004; Kapilashrami & O'Brien, 2012; Pfeiffer & Chapman, 2010). I present in this chapter the examples of key global NGOs to articulate the linkage between transnational capitalism and civil society, and to interrogate the emergence of health as a commodity in the landscape of neoliberal interventionism. What are the consequences of NGO hegemony in the realm of health? What are the problem configurations that are foregrounded in conceptualizing health through the lens of the civil society–market linkage? The choice of these limited set of NGOs is meant to give you an in-depth understanding of the logics of the market that are circulated within the NGO frames, and I invite you to engage with this critical lens in looking at NGOs working in the domain of health.

Democracy Promotion, Neoliberalism, and NGOs

The historical origin of civil society is intertwined with conceptualizations of capitalism and the free market and core assumptions about the role of the individual amid the relationships between the state and the market (Dutta, 2008; Petras, 1997, 1999). Civil society is intertwined with capitalism, closely tied to the economic sphere and connected to the idea that growth in trade and commerce would bring people together in communication and exchange, thus creating spaces for the development of universal codes of human behavior and communication (Frevert, 2005). Frevert (2005, p. 65) posits:

> Civil society was thus built on top of a free market economy, in which its members were support to participate as producers and consumers. But their qualifications as citizens were not restricted to economic achievement, cooperation and consumption. Rather, political philosophy reiterated the complex function of the traditional marketplace as a sphere of economic exchange, social encounter and political debate. In this sense, civil society was devised as a space where citizens could meet in order to socialize with their fellow citizens, to exchange ideas and discuss issues of common concern, to form political opinions.

The key interpretive frames that emerge prominently in neoliberal organizing originate in these early ideas of civil society, built on the notion that as trade and commerce increased, increasing numbers of people would come in close association with each other and this would call for more universal codes of communication and behavior realized through associations in civil society. Free market, intertwined with the conceptualization of the free individual liberated by the market, lies as a foundational principle of civil society.

In a theoretical move predicated on Eurocentric notions of universal progress from a primitive or medieval state of social organization to forms of civilized associations between free and independent citizens participating in the market, the understanding of civil society is predicated on racist interpretive frame that marks the "other" as primitive and outside the realm of civility, and therefore the subject of colonial "civilizing" missions, which were in essence violent, undemocratic, and threatening to human health. Inherent then in the very conceptualization of civil society is a "communicative inversion" that is both paradoxical and threatening to human health. Connecting the circulation of the "civil society" and "democracy" tropes embedded in the imperial agenda marketed as development to the later manifestations of neoliberalism is vital in understanding the ways in which dominant meanings of civil society were intrinsic to the global spread of neoliberal governmentality (Petras, 1997, 1999). Civil society, as spaces for representation of community voices, has been co-opted to serve the agendas of top-down development, often carrying out specific development projects designed by donors. Public opposition to the large-scale and inequitable structures imposed by neoliberal interventions is co-opted into the funding structures of civil society. In his critique of neoliberalism, Harvey (2005,

p. 78) notes, "Non-governmental and grassroots organizations (NGOs and GROs) have also grown and proliferated under neoliberalism, giving rise to the belief that opposition mobilized outside the state apparatus and within some separate entity called 'civil society' is the powerhouse of oppositional politics and social transformations."

U.S. democracy promotion efforts have been carried out on the premise of creating secure spaces for U.S. businesses abroad under the logic of the free market (Petras, 1997, 1999). This emphasis on democracy promotion at the turn of the neoliberal experiment is well captured in U.S. state funding of democracy promotion efforts in the form of the National Endowment for Democracy during the Reagan administration (Petras, 1997, 1999). U.S.-funded development interventions, primarily supported by USAID, have been carried out in the form of promoting media institutions, media structures, and associations, as well as NGOs. The democracy promotion agenda then has been integral to the support for the power elite in nation-states in the global South to assert the U.S. imperial agenda. Such covert forms of imperial penetration, couched in the rhetoric of democracy and civil society promotion, I argue, is fundamentally threatening to human health by fostering conditions that weaken local economies, minimize job opportunities, weaken collective bargaining rights, and weaken the social and public health provisions of the welfare state (Dutta, 2008).

Petras (1997, 1999) observes that in the context of Latin America, in the face of the increasing organizing of social movements resisting the neoliberal model, the United States, the European governments, and WB increased their funding for local NGOs carrying out self-help, popular education, and skills training projects. NGO activities offered Band-Aids in the backdrop of the large-scale job loss, low-paid work, weakened labor regulations, inundation of the local market with cheap imports, and extracting external debt payment that devastated communities. Development projects emerged as outlets for channeling community participation and for co-opting resistive leadership in local communities.

Democracy Promotion and Health Consequences

One of the earliest neoliberal experiments introduced in Chile was accompanied by the U.S.-sponsored multipronged support for local elite NGOs that would promote the opening up of Chile along with clandestine support for the coup organized by Augusto Pinochet to overthrow the popularly elected Sandinista government in Chile, framed in the narrative of democracy promotion. The creation of a space for propping up neoliberal hegemony was achieved through the deployment of violence, thus directly threatening the health and well-being of Chileans. As the oppressions carried out by the Pinochet regime continued building, popular resistance to the regime started formulating strategies of transformation. The United States co-opted this growing popular resistance through the funding of elite NGOs that pushed neoliberal policies and actively thwarted popular resistance against neoliberal policies (Petras, 1997; Robinson, 1996a, 1996b).

Neoliberal policies introduced in Chile privileged the Chilean elite while simultaneously marginalizing the Chilean poor. Economic knowledge linked with the rhetoric of liberty and democracy was deployed within a broader framework of violence and authoritarianism, enabled by the powerful role of elite NGOs funded by U.S. structures in facilitating the opening up of markets (Petras, 1997). Through funding structures framed in the narrative of development and through the participation of NGOs, the United States funneled money into Chile to consolidate power in the hands of the elite and simultaneously curb popular resistance. Further, the elite networks funded by the United States were instrumental in carrying out further the neoliberal reforms that were initially introduced by the Pinochet regime (Robinson, 1996a, 1996b).

The use of violence therefore was intrinsic to the paradigm of neoliberalism introduced into Chile, with the violent suppression of popular democratic participation serving as the opening of the stage for a system of governance that paradoxically sells itself under the promise of democracy. Violence worked precisely to open up the state to the market and to create conditions for the first global experiment on neoliberalization to be carried out in Chile, marrying the agendas of the Chilean elite with the agendas of TNCs. U.S.-style democracy promotion was thus intrinsically connected with the U.S. imperial agenda of opening up markets for U.S.-based corporations. The coup led to the death of over five thousand civilians and to the disappearance of over sixty-five hundred Chilean citizens. The subsequent reign of terror carried out by the Pinochet regime led to the further loss of life in Chile.

Here, threats to health were integral to the direct forms of violence that were constituted in the neoliberal project. Essential to the neoliberal project was the disruption of health, and NGOs emerged as key actors in this process, collaborating globally to pry open markets and to destabilize popular participation, simultaneously working actively toward promoting the further liberalization of Chile. Violence was enacted on the bodies of Chilean citizens under the aegis of democracy promotion efforts sponsored by the United States, working paradoxically to minimize the opportunities for broad-based popular participation in democratic processes that resist neoliberalism (Dutta, 2008). In understanding the threats to health posed by neoliberal interventionism, it is therefore important to highlight the important role of NGOs as structures for promoting neoliberal policies, couched within the language of democracy promotion. Similar violations of health are witnessed in the contexts of U.S. democracy promotion efforts in the Philippines and Nicaragua. More recently, in the contexts of Iraq and Afghanistan, U.S. military interventions have been justified and framed under the logics of promoting democracy, unleashing tremendous forms of violence on civilian populations. NGOs have been essential to the efforts of democracy promotion that ironically have formed the bedrock of these violent interventions, creating new grounds for remaking societies in mirror images of the empire and its capitalist imaginations.

NED has acted as a catalyst in diffusing U.S. values of the free market, narrated under the logic of democracy promotion, across global spaces. NED, with the status of an NGO, has received its major funding from USAID under the umbrella of democracy promotion, and has, in turn, emerged as the channel for disseminating U.S. money and ideology into target countries through elite-owned NGOs in these countries that are aligned with the U.S. agendas of free market promotion. Democracy in this sense is performed as "free elections" with competition among elite actors in these local spaces that are in line with the ideology of the free market. Naming this form of democracy promotion polyarchy, Robinson (1996a) suggests that U.S. democracy promotion efforts have been directed at establishing rule by the power elite in target countries, and simultaneously undermining popular democracy that is driven by the participation of the people in processes of structural transformation. In Chile, Venezuela, Nicaragua, and Cuba, for example, NED efforts have been directed at funding local elite NGOs and media structures that serve as instruments of U.S. propaganda (Robinson, 1996a, 1996b). The public relations functions for transnational hegemony performed by the local NGOs is tied to the active promotion of the free market ideology reframed as democracy.

Democracy promotion thus is tied to the forms of economic reform that in turn produce large-scale impoverishment of the poor while at the same time concentrating resources in the hands of the power elite. The articulation of democracy in this sense acts as a front for the violence that in essence is one of the most powerful predictors of human health (or absence of it). Communicative inversion, depicted in the promises of development and community building, sells the narrative of self-help and community participation even as participation serves as a conduit for carrying out a top-down global agenda. The structural violence produced by neoliberal reforms and through the enabling functions of NGOs, particularly across the global South and the spaces of the South amid the global North, produces a variety of negative health effects. For instance, within the United States, in the context of the financial crisis, large sections of working families were left unemployed or with low wages. The NGO sector, working within the established power structures, offers individualized entrepreneurial solutions to these inequalities and health threats, foreclosing opportunities for transformative politics.

Inequalities, NGOs, and Health

NGOs have played a pivotal role in the circulation and large-scale adoption of the neoliberal frame of global organizing, often aligned with the agendas of WB in restructuring health care systems as private systems of delivery (Campbell, 2014; Forte, 2014; Harvey, 2005). Depicting the welfare recipient as a threat to the structure of neoliberal governance built on the conceptualization of the self-serving individual, NGOs rearticulate the image of the passive poor that is transformed by NGO activities into the participant in entrepreneurial networks, community activities, and self-help groups administered by the NGOs. The image of the brown/black child in fundraising NGO campaigns is the site of NGO action, simultaneously erasing the agency of the poor in the global South and co-opting/erasing the opportunities for participation of the poor in processes of social change and structural transformation. The image of the poor recipient, circulated in the pamphlets, brochures, and Facebook campaigns organized by the NGO sector, becomes the dominant image of fundraising, placing the power of decision making and problem solving into the hands of NGO managers and NGO workers. The narrative of need across the global South however remains unaccounted for in neoliberal structures, with minimal attention paid to evaluating the actual performance of NGOs, the delivery of the services, and the actual meeting of the needs of the underserved communities across the global South.

Beyond their hegemonic functions as organizations delivering support and services to the poor, NGOs occupy key functions in global structures shaping the interpretive frames and meaning frameworks around global governance. In their advocacy functions, NGOs are integral to the production of neoliberal knowledge, offering neoliberal frames around key global frames. The World Economic Forum (WEF), an organization that facilitates the coming together of the global power structures under one umbrella, is an example of the power exerted by NGOs in shaping global agendas. These agendas, often directed by those in positions of power, emerge as agendas of asserting and recycling class power. Civil society, as an accessory to the private sector, collaborates with the private sector in developing advocacy mechanisms for further privatization of global resources, often by selling the very stories and images of poverty that have been produced by neoliberal policies. The image of the "needy" is integral to the fundraising efforts of NGOs, who circulate promotional materials depicting specific communities in need across the global South as strategies for generating resources for NGO operations and activities.

One of the consequences of the SAPs, facilitated and often carried out by elite global NGOs in the global South, has been the rise of inequalities across the various sectors of the globe, both across nation-states as well as within nation-states. NGOs often work toward erasing the structurally transformative opportunities of community participation that seek to address the underlying causes of these inequalities, instead drawing attention to the delivery of specific solutions through individual participation. Noting the role of NGOs as power elites in health and development discourse that profit from the channeling of development and private funds, it is worthwhile to attend to the specific role of health-based NGOs in restructuring health care delivery process.

The functions of NGOs within the neoliberal framework is in delivering specific services and meeting needs that are not met by the reformed state structures. The funding structures of NGOs by donors keeps the NGOs directed toward satisfying donor dictates and frameworks. Within the landscape of global inequalities fostered by neoliberal organizing, NGOs work toward furthering neoliberal agendas of privatization and simultaneously participating in a variety of agendas that weaken state structures. As we will see in the next section, local community participation is co-opted under the managerial structures of NGOs and often under community-based participatory partnerships that co-opt the local community into the folds of the privatizing agenda, diffusing community resistance, community participation in transformative politics, and opportunities for collective mobilization in processes of social change.

Health, NGOs, and the Market

NGOs have been instrumental in establishing the global hegemony of the market, accomplishing their instrumentalist agendas through the linkages they offer between development and health. Development interventions emerge as sites of privatization, often realized through public–private partnerships.

Health and the Market

As we have seen earlier, democracy promotion initiatives constitute the face of dissemination of neoliberal interventions, with the dominant understanding of democracy being constituted under the language of the free market. Health is tied to democratic possibilities as constrained within the framework of the market, understood through the lens of the market. Democracy serves as a trope for neutralizing the market and for making it essential to the organizing of health care. Private corporations emerge on the landscape of health as potential solutions, working hand in hand with NGOs in solving problems of health. Public–private partnerships configure NGOs as key actors in partnering with the private sector to address health problems.

For instance, the World Food Programme (WFP) frames the problem of hunger and the corresponding solutions to hunger in the realm of partnerships with private corporations in catalyzing change through the deployment of food technologies; NGOs are catalyzed within this framework to work with the private sector in addressing food insecurity. For WFP, the win-win proposal for partnering with the private sector offers new opportunities for TNCs to tap into global markets, simultaneously transforming communities and selling the premise of improving livelihoods. Essential here is the role of the NGO sector.

Defining hunger as a health risk, WFP goes on to articulate hunger as a market opportunity under the heading "Engage Consumers" (www.wfp.org/partners/private-sector/why-partner):

> More and more, consumers expect their brands to not only deliver goods and services, but also enable them to do good in the world. By partnering with WFP, brands are seen to be part of the solution to the number one global problem: hunger.

Hunger then emerges as a branding opportunity, as a way to build an image of doing good in the world and thus fulfilling consumer expectations. Brand visibility as a solution to the global problem of hunger therefore also results in additional sales for the commodities that are attached to the programs promoted by the WFP. The image of doing good lies central to the funding logic of the NGOs, working through the articulations of the market to sell health as a commodity, and this generates funding flows both for the NGOs as well as for the TNCs attached to the NGOs.

Similarly, the NGOs working under the framework of Avahan funded by the Gates Foundation work in partnerships with the private sector, privatizing the logic of HIV/AIDS intervention. The reports documenting the Avahan campaign published by the foundation reiterate this logic, highlighting the business model of the intervention and constructing the intervention in economies of scale. The scaling up of the intervention is tied to the scientific logics of management and marketing.

NGOs and Commodities of Health Innovations

Moreover, the commoditization of health through the framework of the market privileges technological solutions to health. Specific problems of health and nutrition are identified in order to push technological solutions, creating new markets for capital. Health solutions are positioned as innovations in the market (www.wfp.org/partners/private-sector/why-partner):

> Tackling social issues from public and private sector perspectives allows partners to approach challenges in new, creative ways—leading to innovation for both WFP and your company. From cutting-edge food technology that combats malnutrition to telecommunication innovations that enables WFP to reach people in far-flung regions with e-vouchers, your company's unique know-how is one key to solving hunger.

Innovation in solving health problems is tied to the innovation for the TNC and to the opportunity for generating profits for the TNC. The commoditization of health is attached to the articulation of health solutions in technologies, thus framing food technology and telecommunications innovations as solutions to hunger. The neoliberalization of health is achieved through the celebration and circulation of technology as a solution, feeding the transnational capitalist economy and simultaneously erasing questions of structural inequality, inequality in distribution of resources, and the role of neoliberalism in constituting the very points of inaccess to resources. Underlying issues of poverty, lack of opportunity, and inaccess remain erased.

Simultaneously, the framing of technology as the solution to health is detached from evidence or documentation of the actual changes in health conditions because of the introduction of the innovation. Technologies such as food fortification by adding nutrients to processed food and biofortification that modifies crops to produce more nutritious yields are positioned as solutions to hunger, simultaneously serving as markets for innovations. Food such as rice and wheat flour are modified, simultaneously erasing the voices of women in the global South who play key roles in producing and preparing food (see Kimura, 2013). Women's needs, resources, and ways of knowing are erased as technologically driven solutions of food commoditized in the market are framed as the solutions to health.

More problematically, in areas such as food technology, the NGO becomes complicit with transnational capital in creating the problem of food insecurity through the commoditization of food resources, privatization of agriculture, minimization of farmer sovereignty, and unequal distribution of food resources in the market logic. Ironically, then, as in the case of food technology, the NGO is part of the problem that constitutes and recycles food insecurity although it operates fundamentally under the framework of solving food insecurity and derives its own brand position through this association.

With the flow of transnational capital in the health sector, NGOs have grown in capacity, often mirroring TNCs in their size and scope, and often offering partner sites for TNCs for market penetration, image building, and building of corporate reputation. Many large NGOs operate as transnational organizations, operating across geographic spaces and having their presence across multiple globally dispersed sites. Through their access to humanitarian issues that leverage the rapidly growing global inequalities brought about by neoliberal interventions, NGOs offer TNCs a global opportunity for building a humanitarian image and for profiting from this humanitarian image. Terms such as *conscious capitalism* become images to be consumed by consumer segments and are sold in the marketplace by NGOs. TNCs associated with global NGOs find access to markets where human health emerges as a branding commodity to be attached to the global image of the NGO as well as of the TNC.

The co-branding of the NGO and of the TNC operates on the site of inequality that has been produced by growth-driven policies constituted under the logic of trickle-down economics. Consider, for instance, the following statement from Unilever on the WFP website:

> "Unilever's support to WFP through Together for Child Vitality means large numbers of school children are being fed nutritious food, educated on matters of hygiene and nutrition and are being given the chance of a better future. And the bonus is that doing this makes our business healthier too." (Paul Polman, Unilever)

The creation of health opportunities for large numbers of school children is tied to the healthier business opportunities for Unilever. Individual health is constituted within corporatized health. Therefore, the poor health and poor nutrition of large numbers of schoolchildren becomes a market opportunity for Unilever, creating a scenario for it to profit, simultaneously disregarding the large-scale inequalities that are generated by the profit-driven logic and the underlying liberalization of infrastructures. The framework of privatization as a solution to lack of nutrition ironically perpetuates the very institutional structures of neoliberalism that cause the inequalities at the first hand. Note here individual-level assumptions of what makes up health and the care of health. The nutritious food that is being packaged under the program is technologically devised food, once again privileging the framework of technological innovation in the free market, tied to the purchasing power of the individual (Phelps, 2012).

Individual Responsibility and the Market

The organizing narrative of neoliberalism imparts meaning to health through the foregrounding of individual responsibility and ownership

(Brown & Baker, 2012). The individualization of health is achieved through the emphasis placed on individual belief, attitudes, and behaviors, with health solutions being directed at inducing individual change (Dutta, 2008). Interventions are directed at promoting ownership of health through concepts such as self-efficacy and empowerment. NGOs emerge in this landscape as the structures for disseminating health services directed at the individual as well as for disseminating health information and communication strategies that would induce positive behavioral change.

As noted earlier, the "Together for Child Vitality" program funded by the WFP is framed within the logics of imparting education to the children about hygiene and nutrition and about giving the children chances for a better future. Embodied in the articulation is the logic of neoliberalism that privileges technologies of health along with an emphasis on individual ownership and simultaneously erases the underlying structural inequities from the discursive space. The localization of health achieved through the NGOs also privileges the framework of individual lifestyle change and individually directed ownership. Consider, for instance, the "Food for Assets" program run by the NGO Mercy Corps and funded by the WFP in Sudan. Here is the definition of the program on the WFP website (www.wfp.org/content/ngo-puts-south-sudanese-work-food):

> An international NGO has been putting people in a drought-stricken area of South Sudan to work, in exchange for food. The new program, called "Food for Assets," is run by Mercy Corps and allows people in an area in Aweil East, in Northern Bahr el Ghazal, to work on projects that benefit their community, in exchange for food. The food is supplied by the United Nations' World Food Program, and the projects locals work on include everything from clearing roads that link local villages to improving irrigation systems on small farms.

Once again, the provision of food as a basic capacity in a resource-deprived sector is tied to work. Individual responsibility and accountability are the key determinants of access to food. Elements of public infrastructure such as improving irrigation systems and clearing roads are introduced into the market logic, to be exchanged with another public welfare function, the provision of basic food necessities in a resource-deprived setting. The logic of neoliberalism works here through the marketization of two public necessities, setting them in opposition to each other in the logic of exchange and thus profiting the NGO in the process. The commoditization of public infrastructures benefits the NGO and its economic structure through the individualization of health.

Consider similarly the Avahan HIV/AIDS campaign in India that is carried out by over one hundred NGOs in India that are funded by the Bill and

Melinda Gates Foundation (see Dutta & Acharya, 2014). Avahan achieves its goal of addressing the risk behaviors of truckers by individualizing the responsibility of sexual behavior and simultaneously erasing the structural contexts of trucking that constitute HIV/AIDS risk. For instance, truckers are educated about the proper use of condoms and about the risks of unsafe sexual behavior. NGOs are deployed to provide educational programs and to distribute condoms. Broader issues of liberalization, the accompanying marginalization of agriculture, and the economic disenfranchisement of rural communities remain absent from the configuration of the campaign and its measures of effectiveness. The document "Avahan—The India AIDS Initiative: The Business of HIV Prevention and Scale" (Avahan, 2008) highlights the role of peer educators in modifying and monitoring individual behavior:

> As part of continuous program improvement, Avahan partners use "micro-planning" as an approach to fine-tune implementation at the grassroots level. Micro-planning involves peer educators gathering detailed, multi-faceted information from "hotspots" (high-risk venues where commercial sex is solicited) to understand the nature of intervention needed. This is followed by systematic, ongoing outreach to the high-risk groups in these venues. Peer educators manage and monitor 25–50 peer members in their assigned group and work about four hours per day. Their activities include sharing prevention information with their colleagues, distributing condoms (and as appropriate needles and syringes), making referrals to clinics and other services, and gathering information on each individual's risk profile, including their vulnerability to violence and their ability to access services. (p. 13)

Concepts of participation, community mobilization, and peer-to-peer outreach are constituted within the broader goals of the campaign to disseminate information and condoms. The participation of peer educators is constructed within the individualization of health, married to the tasks of sharing prevention information, distributing condoms, and gathering risk information on peer members. Individualization therefore is tied not only to information dissemination but also to surveillance.

The frame circulated in the civil society–private sector linkage erases the inequities in distribution of food in spite of the stockpile of food in global sectors of control. Also note that the articulation of the program does not really offer empirical data on the health outcomes of the children, the long-term health impacts of the program, and the specifics of what a better future for the children translates into over the long term. Therefore, the fundamental understanding of human health is shaped by the emphasis on the individual as a participant in the marketplace. In this sense, the idea of democratic participation is deeply intertwined with the commoditization of individual subjectivity, where the acknowledgment of the citizen is tied to his/her ability to participate in the market as a consumer and to his/her position as a property-bearing subject. Health therefore is articulated as a commodity that can be achieved through productive participation in the market, inherently connected to the ownership of capital. For instance, the NGO PATH has played a prominent role in the dissemination of the market logic through its work in the health sector, often framed within the language of democratic participation. Other NGOs emerge as key actors in the promotion of democracy globally, apparently bringing the U.S. values of liberty and freedom in the world. The face of democracy promotion in the global South has been embodied in transnational support for NGOs that have played pivotal roles in the diffusion of imperial notions of democracy shaped by the aspirations of capital and free market.

Managerialism and the NGO Sector

In the example of programs cited above, the WFP works with expert consulting groups such as the Boston Consulting Group to consolidate the decision-making capacities in the hands of a global elite coterie of experts, paying their paychecks by establishing poverty as a problem and further erasing the participatory opportunities for local communities in articulating and owning health solutions and in participating toward community-driven health opportunities. Participation is conceptualized within the dictates of the professional managers that establish objectives, deliverables, and evaluative parameters for projects.

Health emerges in the form of specific portfolios and projects to be handled by program managers and project leads, with definite starting and ending points that are connected to project evaluation. Funding agencies establish the parameters of success, and NGOs operate within these parameters through the deployment of management principles. The Avahan example cited earlier works through the deployment of principles of marketing to the problematization of HIV/AIDS. The solutions therefore are constructed within the framework of marketing. The evaluation of the campaign and the campaign reports reflect the managerial agenda in articulating a business of scale. To run Avahan, a coterie of management consultants are hired and placed in India; management consultants head the team to implement a business model in carrying out the health intervention. Note, for instance, the language of marketing that is integral to the dissemination of condoms to be carried out by NGOs at the local sites:

> Examples of non-traditional outlets include tea and pan shops (tobacco and cigarette shops), roadside restaurants, local all-purpose grocery stores, vending machines at truck stops, and health clinics. This effort is supported by promoting condom normalization through a combination of active mid-media efforts (street theatre, retailer promotions) and mass media campaigns (television, radio, movies, billboards). Over 147,000 outlets stocking condoms have been opened by Avahan in high-risk venues in the four southern states and across the national highways. By the end of 2007 these outlets were selling about 5 million socially marketed condoms per month to men at risk. (Avahan, 2008, p. 15)

Nontraditional channels for disseminating condoms serve as elements of the marketing mix. Condom promotion and normalization through nontraditional channels is positioned as an innovative strategy of distribution. The delivery of health is shaped within the marketing logic of Avahan, with the at-risk groups such as truckers and sex workers intrinsically constructed as the potential markets. The managerialization of health is linked with the profit motives of the elite sectors, turning health into a private sector resource to be exploited in market logics. The large salaries of management consultants and development experts take up significant proportions of resources allocated to health under the aegis of development. Such professionalization of health also then is tied to the economic incentives of the bourgeoisie classes across nation-states who work in the development sector and earn their livings through grants and funding initiatives.

Top-Down Communication, Community Participation

As noted earlier in this chapter, community participation is the new buzzword for donor-driven NGOs. The language of community participation stands as an example of communicative inversion as participation often is co-opted into the very structures of the NGO formations and NGO projects. The community is constituted within the ambits of a preconfigured NGO agenda, and community participation is defined in relationship to this existing agenda. Participatory communication channels therefore become devices for carrying out the top-down goals as designed by experts and conceived by funders. For instance, NGOs working on multiple WB projects are driven toward circulating the WB agenda of free market expansion while at the same time doing so through the language of the community and community participation.

The nature of participation therefore is interpreted as a channel carrying out the objectives of the funding agencies. The community, thus defined as a monolith, becomes the target of top-down expert-driven interventions, with participation emerging as a co-optive channel for securing community buy-in and ownership. The agenda, albeit directed toward the structures of the funding agency, is framed within the broader goals and structures of neoliberalism. The possibilities of community participation in addressing unequal health structures, in challenging the organizing logics of these structures, and in seeking structural transformation are erased from the discursive space.

Negotiating Transparency and Accountability

Amid the calls for greater transparency and accountability issued within the dominant structures of neoliberal governance, the linkages that constitute the relationships between civil society organizations, TNCs, state actors, and knowledge generating bodies such as consulting firms and think tanks remain hidden. The NGO PATH, for instance, is run by leaders who have moved between the for-profit sector, the consulting sector, the human rights sector, and the NGO sector, depicting the revolving door between NGOs and transnational capital. Steve Davis, the president and CEO of PATH, ran the Bill Gates–owned digital media firm Corbis, which had been found to have committed fraud against Infoflows Corporation for stealing intellectual property (Buley, 2010). Similarly, during Davis' stint as the leader of PATH's programs in India, PATH came under the scrutiny of grassroots activists for the violation of informed consent principles alongside criticisms of its relationships with transnational pharmaceutical corporations Merck and GlaxoSmithKline.

NGOs such as PATH depict the problems that are brought about by the large-scale privatization of the bio-sector, with NGOs playing often unclear and problematic roles in opening up markets through bio-investments, framed in the rhetoric of development and improved human health outcomes. Moreover, the techno-scientific language of science is deployed by NGOs within these contexts to obscure questions of accountability, questions asking for evidence, questions interrogating conflicts of interest, and greater calls for transparency. In a process of "communicative erasure," the language of science is actively deployed to silence public discussions of science, the claims of innovation, and questions of effectiveness and side effects.

In the instance of the ongoing protests in India on the violations of bioethics by PATH in the ways in which it did or did not secure informed consent from the girls and their parents in an HPV vaccination project in India, Davis responds in an interview with Timmerman (2010) for Xconomy: "You think about big strategies and PowerPoints and we need more than that to understand what's going on. It translates differently when you deal with bureaucrats, crazy political moves, people dynamics, and state-by-state issues." The unquestionable benefits of science and technology are positioned in opposition to cultural resistance to adaptation. The framing of calls for greater transparency and accountability and interrogation of potential conflicts of interest in the relationship of the NGO with transnational capital are framed as barriers to be overcome, thus erasing opportunities for critical interrogation and dialogue. Moreover, through a process of "communicative inversion," the questions raised by local activists are reframed in a narrative of inequality of access to HPV vaccine, obfuscating the issues of profits, unethical processes in securing consent in clinical trials, and unequal structures of profiting clinical trials in the global South that are raised by activists. Moreover, the discursive portrayal of calls for greater transparency and accountability as reflections of a primitive state formation reproduces the racist tropes of neoliberalism.

On a similar note, in the context of the active advocacy role played by PATH in supporting agricultural biotechnology, with most of the funding coming from the Gates Foundation, it is worthwhile to interrogate the conflicts of interest raised by the investments of the foundation in agrobiotech transnationals such as Monsanto and the mediatizing role played by the NGO in whitewashing these linkages, obscuring them, and rendering them invisible. Accountability therefore needs to be conceptualized in terms of mapping the flow of financial resources and the nature of profit-driven enterprise that pushes the diffusion of bio-commodities through the dissemination role of NGOs. Worth interrogating are the communicative disjunctures between the questions of ethics raised regarding the organizational and leadership structure in PATH and the advocacy role played by the NGO in the global arena, pushing technological innovations to problems of health and development. As PATH champions biotechnology as a solution to problems of human development and health at the WEF, a close reading of the track record would raise critical questions regarding conflicts of interest, past criticisms of intellectual piracy, and references to unethical practices. In the global circuits of power, communicative erasure works consistently to obliterate these critical questions, creating continual opportunity spaces for NGOs to deploy their nonprofit facade of altruism and development to push questionable agendas of transnational capitalism.

NGOs, Corporatization, and Health Risks

In this section, we specifically examine the negative role of NGOs in bringing about health risks through their participation in projects of transnational hegemony that directly threaten human health. NGOs play pivotal roles in greenwashing the image of TNCs and in framing a facade of community development through corporate social responsibility programs. For instance, NGOs serve as the partners in CSR programs of TNCs in the extractive sectors (Padel & Das, 2010). In this function, NGOs minimize the perceived threat around the operations of extractive industries as well as generate positive public opinion around the TNCs. In other instances, NGOs actively participate in producing information that detract attention away from the health-threatening functions of TNCs. Similarly, NGOs often detract the focus away from the underlying structural contexts of health disparities, instead foregrounding individualized solutions in the language of empowerment.

NGOs and Health Privatization

NGOs have played key roles in economic restructuring processes globally, particularly in the transformation of public health infrastructures into privatized modes of delivery (Pfeiffer, 2003). With their funding structures driven by donor agendas, these NGOs have become global conduits for imposing top-down agendas of structural adjustment (Kamat, 2004; Loevinsohn & Harding, 2005; Turshen, 1999), transforming the health sector into market opportunities for managed care, insurance agencies, and health management organizations. In carrying out the agendas of privatizing health care, NAFTA and the Free Trade Area of the Americas (FTAA) pushed health care markets for U.S.-based insurance corporations in Latin America (Waitzkin, 2011). NGOs are integral to neoliberal restructuring of health care, with the increasing funding and staffing of professional NGOs as sites of delivery of health care in the backdrop of the weakening of public health infrastructures, resources, and services (Schuller, 2009; Timmer, 2010).

The dominant narrative supporting the privatization of health care is constituted under the logic of efficiency, pointing to inefficiencies and corruption in the private sector as barriers to the effective delivery of health care. The facade offered by the not-for-profit narrative of NGOs played a key public relations role in the privatization of health care. Development organizations such as USAID play pivotal roles in organizing the privatizing of health care through so-called development programs that are directed at and channeled through NGOs (Armada, Muntaner & Navarro, 2001). In countries such as Bolivia, U.S.-funded development funds directed at NGOs have been pivotal to the shaping of public opinion and to policy advocacy work that has enabled the privatization of health care. Moreover, NGOs, mostly comprising elite leadership classes funded by donor agencies, are integral to the imposition of top-down agendas in communities, often positioned in the language of participatory health management.

The weakening of public health services and the disruptions in public health delivery by neoliberal adjustments have weakened the delivery of preventive services, the absence of basic care, and the lack of coordinated state-driven infrastructures at addressing public health needs. The communicative promises of efficient and effective health care are far from being realized, with health care tied to the agendas of profiteering (Waitzkin, 2011).

NGOs and Land Acquisition

As TNCs have expanded their global reach, one of the ongoing areas of TNC control has been the mineral wealth sector. NGOs have emerged as key actors in the market of mineral resources as raw materials in the global economy, setting up opportunities for new resources to be harvested across global sites and often threatening to displace subaltern communities, working with the corporate social responsibility (CSR) outfits of private corporations to minimize dissent and to co-opt the opportunities for subaltern participation. As communities from the margins in the global South are displaced from their ancestral homes, CSR programs work hard to manage image and offer a positive branding strategy in their linkages with NGOs. The cultural erasure of subaltern communities and the health threats that are intertwined with these erasures form the bases for civil society–market relationships.

NGOs carrying out health promotion programs, for instance, become the facade for public relations for these extractive industries, simultaneously erasing the fundamental threats to health that are posed by the extractive industries. In such instances, NGOs create a human face for the oppressive forces of extractive TNCs that whitewash over the health threats and threats to dignity of displaced communities. The materiality of exploitation is hidden under the notion of health improvements through health promotion programs.

NGOs create opportunities for engagement with schools, community projects, and health projects to narrate a positive story that detracts from the reality of land acquisition, displacement, and fundamental threats to health that are posed by transnational extractive industries such as mining corporations (Padel & Das, 2010). For example, even as an NGO working with a mining TNC works to create a hospital to create a positive image, it erases the very threats to health that are produced by the pollution and displacement generated by the mining operation. In India, for instance, the NGO Pratham served as the face of the mining giant Vedanta as it went about developing mining operations in the Niyamgiri Hills of Odisha. Similarly, at a global level, the international NGO Survival International gained tremendous visibility in articulating a politics of indigenous resistance to global mining operations by narrating solidarity with indigenous communities even as Survival draws much of its international funding from transnational hegemony. Similarly, the global NGO Association for India's Development drew its branding from associating the movement of the Dongria Kondh resisting the mining operations by Vedanta in the Niyamgiri Hills, while simultaneously drawing financial resources from Vedanta and from other TNCs. These NGOs, constituted within the very logics of neoliberalism that constitute the hegemony of transnational capital, participate on strategic "communicative inversions," simultaneously serving the logics of transnational capital, offering branding opportunities for transnational capitalism, and putting forth the face of resistance, transformation, social change, democracy, and grassroots participation.

In their functions in carrying out community relations functions for their corporate funders, NGOs deliver the community interface for engagement. The facade of community activities carried out by NGOs serve as the organizing logics for co-opting, manipulating, and subverting community agency. NGOs in such contexts of land acquisition also act as information-gathering tools for gathering relevant data on the potential sites of resistance to the displacement agendas. Additional community relations activities are further driven toward co-opting this agenda.

NGOs and Pollution

Globally, NGOs perform key functions in greenwashing the image of TNCs that generate economic revenues through processes of production that threaten human health through their harmful effects on the environment. CSR programs run by TNCs polluting the environment achieve positive images for the TNCs through funded NGO activities that attach the TNC with a positive image (Burton, 2007). Through the funding structures that are integral to the logic, organizing, and functioning of NGOs, especially large transnational NGOs, TNCs seek out branding opportunities that contribute to a positive image.

Strategically communicating an image that draws on narratives of sustainability and eco-friendliness, TNCs support NGO-driven projects in order to build community ties, secure community participation, co-opt community resistance, and create brand associations that leverage environmental consciousness as a segmenting and targeting variable. In his analysis of TNC funding of NGOs as a public relations tactic, Burton (2007) points to the strategic deployment of public relations as community engagement to co-opt NGOs into the folds of TNCs. NGOs working within the realm of development often offer the neutral image that is needed by TNCs to circulate particular forms of knowledge claims. Development projects such as building schools, empowering girls, and building water resources draw attention away from the environmental pollution being caused by the TNCs.

For example, in the context of the large-scale deforestation produced by the palm oil industry, especially in tropical rain forests such as those in Southeast Asia, major palm-oil-using TNCs such as Unilever fund "clean" NGO projects and articulate a commitment to deforestation even as they participate in the production of knowledge with conflicts of interest such as the high carbon stock forest study (SumofUs, n.d.). The definition of what constitutes "high carbon stock" forests is central to the deforestation processes as it delineates the guidelines for forests that can be cut for the purposes of palm oil production. NGOs offer the neutral face for channeling the money into communicative processes that generate knowledge and shape knowledge claims (Burton, 2007). NGOs such as the World Wildlife Fund (WWF) emerge as channels for greenwashing the environmentally unsustainable actions of TNCs, often formulated in the form of locally sustainable projects embodying NGO–TNC partnerships (Burton, 2007).

In the face of public resistance toward and criticism of TNCs, NGOs emerge as conduits for articulating knowledge claims directed at shaping public opinion and simultaneously developing branding strategies that lend credibility to TNCs through joint projects. Let's take for instance the Unilever-funded partnership between Unilever and WWF in launching a nonprofit organization called the Marine Stewardship Council (MSC) that would offer accreditation to "sustainable fishery" in the face of the growing resistance in the 1990s against unsustainable fishing that threatened Unilever frozen fish brands such as Bird's Eye and Igloo (Burton, 2007). MSC launched an accreditation process, and in one of its initial initiatives, granted New Zealand–based consultancy firm SGS Product and Process Certification for certifying the New Zealand hoki fish. The accreditation label offered by MSC to the hoki fishing industry in New Zealand, supplying hoki to Frozen Fish International, a subsidiary of Unilever, in spite of criticism from environmental groups in New Zealand about the unsustainable practices of the fishery that led to an estimated drowning of more than fifty-six hundred seals between 1989 and 1998, created new markets in the United States, Europe, and Australia for hoki fish and gave the hoki fish market advantage over other whitefish. The accreditation process and accreditation label offered by MSC depict the interplay of the interests of TNCs and transnational NGOs in generating branding claims that underlie competitive advantage, market share, and market leadership. NGOs thus become the instruments of the market, functioning as instruments of branding. This branding function of NGOs becomes evident in an internal e-mail exchange between the chief executive of WWF New Zealand, J. O. Breese, and the head of WWF International, Claude Martin, expressing reservations about the accreditation (cited in Burton, 2007, p. 166):

> There are some sensitive issues, e.g., 1000 fur seals killed per year, by-catch of seabirds and maintaining the fish stock. These could potentially "blow up" in the media and be very damaging internationally to WWF, MSC, and SGS.

Transnational NGOs such as WWF and Action Aid depend upon large sums of money to run their operations, and thus are driven toward funding structures to run their organizational operations. Particularly worth noting are the high pay structures of NGO staff and the managerial logic that percolates into NGOs, removed from the everyday lived experiences of the target communities that NGOs frame as recipients of interventions. The political economy of NGOs is constituted in the realm of knowledge production that casts communities as passive, underdeveloped, and in need for the interventions carried out by the NGOs. NGOs such as Christian Aid draw upon the narrative of the primitive "other" to constitute their funding structures, thus recycling the tropes of missionary intervention reframed in the language of the free market, empowerment, self-help, and therapeutic messaging that aims to uplift recipient audiences into higher levels of self and collective efficacy. Moreover, knowledge produced by NGOs is often specifically directed toward silencing alternative articulations in the backdrop of the functions of TNCs. The NGO in such instances offers the facade for objective knowledge, dislocating the source of the message and reframing the message within an activist narrative in order to whitewash the underlying materiality.

NGOs and Bioprofits

NGOs such as PATH are integral to the prevailing global model of health driven by bioprofits. The realm of the "bio" is also the arena for profiteering, turning bodies, genes, and life into exploitable resources in interconnected networks of global profiteering. The nonprofit face of the NGO sector works in managing resources, securing biomaterials, coordinating the flow of these materials, developing testing sites for randomized controlled trials, carrying out studies, identifying markets, and disseminating health products in these markets, and in channeling health resources into networks of profiteering. For instance, in the realm of the dissemination of the Bt.

technology as a development solution, NGOs served as the front for a number of dissemination projects, hiding the corporate motive of profiteering within a narrative of development and social change.

In most instances, the relationships of the NGOs with the networks of profiteering remain obscured. Leadership structures of powerful NGOs are intertwined with leadership structures of private corporations and foundations, thus playing out the corporate agenda in articulations of knowledge claim. The NGO emerges as the face of science, turning science into a resource for profiteering. NGOs occupy key roles in public–private partnerships, especially in the realm of delivery of bio-solutions that are delivered in exchange for grants that fund NGO projects.

Resisting Free Markets: Alternative Rationalities of Democracy

The possibilities of achieving health in the subaltern sectors of the globe are tied to the co-constructions with subaltern communities in the global margins that voice alternative meanings of health, grounded in everyday negotiations of life. The materiality of the lived experiences of subaltern communities, narrated through the experiences of health, offers an axis for entering into discourses of health. Through their everyday struggles in negotiating health, in protecting their resources of health that are threatened by the onslaught of the market and the accompanying development logics, and through their participation in grassroots processes of organizing, subaltern communities participate in transforming the politics of health. In this section, I argue that the spheres of everyday politics, intersecting with the markers of privilege in civil society, offer opportunities of structural transformation.

Strategies of Resistance

Even as this chapter points toward the role of NGOs in circulating the health-threatening logics perpetuated by TNCs, NGOs also serve as sites of resistance to the politics of co-optation catalyzed by transnational hegemony, working through possibilities of solidarity with subaltern communities. The communicative character of resistance is transformative, working to foster communicative equality and to counter the communicative inversions that are integral to neoliberal hegemony. Fostering spaces for transparent communication and evidence-based information sharing is an entry point to the politics of social change. Similarly, connecting health communication to local processes of organizing fosters opportunities for transforming the co-optation of community participatory spaces as instruments of neoliberalism.

Spaces for Alternative Imaginations

NGOs, as organizational structures that exist outside the realms of the market and the state, also offer openings for alternative imaginations even as much of the funded NGO work draws from elite networks of transnational capitalism that shape the agendas of NGOs. To engage creatively with new possibilities, participatory platforms fostered by NGOs need to be held accountable to community expectations, community needs, and community imaginations of solutions. The dominant framework of NGO accountability to national and global private–public donors needs to be resisted by a framework of accountability that turns toward subaltern communities at the margins of the neoliberal reforms. The donor-driven organizing space of NGO work is actively resisted with a vision for NGO work that is grounded in community activism, transformative politics, and community voices. The managerial structures of NGOs that have transformed NGO work as the aspirations for a professional class are reworked into a new narrative of NGO work that is driven by activism, community voices, and transformative agendas of global social change. Social change is thus defined structurally in a dialectical–dialogical relationship with the dominant organizing structures, drawing upon a range of communication strategies from dialogue to direct confrontation to define new possibilities for participation.

Spaces for Solidarity

Amid the neoliberal structuring of NGOs as catalysts of privatization processes, the spaces for global networking enabled by globalization processes also foster opportunities for resistance on a global platform. NGOs resisting mining operations in global contexts demonstrate the important role NGOs can play in transforming neoliberal processes of exploitation of local communities, fostering spaces for listening to community voices. However, within the context of resistance to mining, Padel and Das (2010) depict the interplay of resistance and co-optation of NGOs, with NGO funding being integral to the co-optation of NGOs. To the extent that NGOs remain donor driven and are directed by their funders in the community work they carry out, their agendas are likely to be co-opted by the private sector and by powerful actors of globalization politics. The realm of accountability driven toward funders and driven by funder agendas fosters a structure that is not directed to subaltern communities in the global South.

However, a strategic response that is critically aware and reflexive about funding sources and is committed to building solidarity with the poor and the underserved can offer an entry point for transforming the health-threatening effects of neoliberalism. In such processes of local solidarity, the sphere of solidarity is turned toward the communities in the margins. The NGO then becomes situated in the context of its commitment to community norms, community expectations, and community voices. Solidarity, as a long-term partnership with communities, fosters a communicative context of participatory communication that is guided by community interpretations, understandings of problems, and participation in developing solutions. Therefore, it is vital to turn the sphere of accountability to local community voices and community participation, inverting the dominant structures of neoliberalism within which NGOs are constituted. Turning the possibilities of accountability to communities fosters spaces for delivering policies and programs that are rooted in community imaginations, community interpretations, and community frameworks of problems and solutions.

Conclusion

In this chapter, I have argued that the dominant organizing framework for global health operates on the formulation of civil society as an integral player in the processes of privatization of health. The role of NGOs is constituted within this dominant framework as one of carrying out the agendas of funders, driven by top-down expertise, often co-opting local community participation to offer a whitewashed facade to the neoliberal agenda. The possibilities of transforming the NGO sector come from the consideration of the role of resistance as an organizing framework for the practice of NGO work. Moreover, when the realms of accountability are shifted in the direction of communities, NGOs become more accountable to the communities they serve. Community participation as a transformative practice works toward holding NGOs accountable in the global structure.

CHAPTER SIX

HEALTH AS SECURITY: CRISIS, SURVEILLANCE, AND MANAGEMENT

The globalization of economies has produced accelerated patterns of movements of capital, goods, services, materials, and labor, simultaneously resulting in the accelerated production and circulation of anxieties constituted around these movements. Neoliberal organizing of health manifests itself in the development and deployment of surveillance, management, and coordination networks that see health primarily in the realm of threats posed by diseases dispersed through global networks, networks of bioterror, emerging infectious diseases, and biowarfare (Salinsky, 2002). The response of health systems therefore is formulated in the form of network structures of biodefense and homeland security, performing functions of surveillance, information gathering, and information dissemination, constituted around the economic logics of growth and efficiency. The protection of the economic opportunities of globalization becomes the function of public health systems formulated in the narrative of geosecurity and implemented in the form of programs controlled by the police-military complex within structures of biodefense, biosecurity and geosecurity.

With this emphasis on security, the mandate for health depicts continuity with colonial implementations of public health administration to manage erstwhile colonies, increasingly being set within the military metaphor of health, turning health into a geosecurity threat for the new configurations of empire, and therefore, deploying military interventions to address health issues. Consider the following depiction in a report issued by the U.S. National Intelligence Council (NIC) that offers a picture of the global health threats posed by infectious diseases:

> New and reemerging infectious diseases will pose a rising global health threat and will complicate U.S. and global security over the next twenty years. These diseases will endanger U.S. citizens at home and abroad, threaten U.S. armed forces deployed overseas, and exacerbate social and political instability in key countries and regions in which the United States has significant interests. (Gordon, 2000)

The protection of human health is seen as a function of the military, tied to the goals of defending global capitalism against the threats to health and reflecting the colonial undertones of health containment measures deployed by the instruments of empire. In this instance of the report published by the NIC, knowledge about health is constituted in the realm of intelligence gathering to protect the interests of national security of the United States.

Framed as threats to the health of citizens at home and abroad and to the health of the armed forces deployed overseas, infectious diseases are seen as contributors to social and political instability in key strategic regions of significant value to the United States. International relations are understood in the language of security, casting interpenetrating networks as targets of surveillance and management. The portrayal of infectious diseases as threats to geosecurity deploys valuable health resources into the hands of the military, placing the power of disease management under military structures and framing the responses to disease in military interpretations. Moreover, the juxtaposition of epidemic narratives amid narratives of war and bioterror heighten the concerns for geosecurity, foregrounding and necessitating a variety of military response strategies (Aaltola, 2012).

The interpenetrating relationship between health and the military constitute one element of the consolidation of power in the hands of the global elite achieved through neoliberal transformations. The military emerges as a global organizational structure for the management of health, simultaneously justifying the deployment of resources to the military and the deployment of military strategies to address health issues. This emphasis on the military framed within the realm of protecting geostrategic interests constructs health in the realm of threats, simultaneously erasing questions of fundamental human rights to health. Similarly, in the president's Emergency Plan for AIDS Relief, a significant proportion of resources are housed in the military in order to deploy military-to-military interventions within the broader umbrella of protecting the geostrategic interests of the United States. Consider, for instance, the workings of the U.S. Africa Command to address HIV/AIDS prevention as a security threat in Africa.

> The U.S. Africa Command (AFRICOM) is the result of an internal reorganization of the U.S. military command structure, creating one administrative headquarters that answers to the Secretary of Defense and is responsible for U.S. military relations with 53 African countries. AFRICOM recognizes that HIV/AIDS has an enormous impact on economic and political stability across the continent, and, by degrading military medical readiness, weakens the national security of individual countries. HIV/AIDS programming will be a key component of AFRICOM's security cooperation and humanitarian assistance activities. (www.pepfar.gov/about/agencies/c19397.htm)

Critical to the deployment of a militarized form of governance in addressing health is the consolidation of power within elite structures, working through militarized systems of governance to control disease to protect the economic interests of the status quo. The military, as an instrument of power and control, functions within the narratives of security cooperation and humanitarian assistance activities to assert its power and control in global governance. Intelligence gathering emerges as an instrument for the generation of data to secure and protect zones of economic function. This gathering of targeted intelligence and the deployment of targeted interventions becomes particularly critical within the context of maintaining open zones of communication and economic exchange within the neoliberal structuring of economic relationships. Knowledge and technical interventions in this sense are constituted amid the paradoxical agenda of needing to protect boundaries and at the same time ensuring transnational spaces of movement of capital, labor, services, materials, and markets. In this chapter, we closely interrogate the meanings that circulate around the militarization of health, and attend to the communicative processes through which the militarization of health is achieved. The surveillance of spaces and the militarization of responses, I argue, are continuous with colonial logics of controlling spaces in distant locales of imperial governance, and are discontinuous from the colonial forms of governance because of the paradoxes of networked flows in neoliberal governance.

Militarization, Incarceration, and Threats to Health

The militarization of global organizing refers to the large-scale deployment of resources toward the military as a framework of global governance. Defense corporations constitute some of the most profitable segments of transnational capitalism. For many of the largest democracies globally, defense budgets are shaped in the realm of public–private partnerships, connecting public resources to new market opportunities for profiteering through the circulation of narratives of terrorism and threats to geosecurity. More investment in new technologies of war is the consistent call for global crisis management, offered as the solution or threats to geosecurity, freedom, and economic progress.

War and Health

One of the most fundamental forms of threat to human health is war (Loyd, 2009). The health effects of war are witnessed across global sites of violence, from Gaza to Iraq to Afghanistan to Lebanon and Syria. Wars, through the effectiveness of new and more advanced technologies, produce widespread devastation, from deaths of civilians to adverse health impacts in civilian populations, to deaths of soldiers and poor health outcomes of soldiers serving in wars. As witnessed in the recent Israeli attacks on Gaza, wars often directly impact the health of women and children. By the time of writing this chapter, Israel defense forces had killed fourteen hundred civilians in Gaza, with 435 of these civilians being children. As in the case of the recent Israeli occupation of Gaza, sites of healing such as hospitals become targets of military attacks, thus fundamentally disrupting the very fabric of health, erasing symbolically and materially possibilities of healing.

With the increasing sophistication of new technologies of war, wars emerge as sites of tremendous violence, achieved through the deployment of sophisticated technologies. In the post–Cold War period, the language of war is intrinsically tied to the language of security, with justifications for war voiced in narratives of fighting terrorism and fostering secure spaces. War also serves as a mechanism of resource extraction, for instance, being strategically deployed in regions with mineral resources in order to enable exploitative patterns of extraction. The military interventions, for instance, carried out by Israel in the West Bank secures spaces of production and profiteering for transnational corporations such as SodaStream, the security company G4S, and the technology company Hewlett-Packard. Consider, for instance, the following articulation by Goldberg (2009, p. 347):

> Rogue states are those that have "proved" for a variety of reasons that they cannot be controlled or managed by the "soft power" of debt regulation, structural adjustment, persuasive investment, and ideological rationalization in the new global scheme of neoliberalism. These are the sorts of states identified by George Bush as representing the "axis of evil": Iran, Iraq, Syria, Palestine, North Korea, Venezuela, Cuba. If the euro mimesis at the heart of racial mixture holds out to those engaged in the mixing a possibility of entering even a diminished whiteness, then rogue states are states (where properly states at all) of various sorts of non-whiteness, structurally understood. Mutant states, they are states, that is, of anti-whiteness, which is to say, anti-Americanism. In short, of debilitated racial definition. Inferior, savage, untrustworthy.

Communication plays a pivotal role in fostering neocolonial interventions within neoliberal global structures. The "other," manifested as a threat to global geosecurity, often framed as a threat to a homogeneous Western civilization and its modern ways, must be contained and controlled through invasions. The narratives of contagion, contamination, and spiraling threat are drawn from portrayals of epidemics as justifications for war as strategies of decontamination and containment. For instance, Aaltola (2012) draws attention to the circulation of tropes of epidemics, bioterror, and biological threats in U.S. official narratives building up to the Iraq war.

The language of security therefore becomes a facade for the colonial extraction of resources, feeding neoliberal structures of power in global networks. Once again, within the context of wars, the linkage between neoliberalism and violence becomes worthwhile to explore. As noted in Chapter One in the book, the U.S. support for a violent coup in Chile and the military support of the Pinochet dictatorship to Chile served as the backdrop for the first neoliberal experiment (Harvey, 2003, 2005, 2006). More recently, the U.S. invasion of Iraq served as a pretext for redoing the Iraqi economy in the logics of free market economics. States resisting the free market structures of neoliberalism are portrayed as states opposed to the ways of the free world. Covert and overt wars are used as strategies to reconfigure economies resisting the global neoliberal structure, incorporating them into the global free market structure by positioning the free market as the beacon of freedom and liberty.

Global supplies in arms and instruments of violence constitute the fabric of the war-military industry, thus constituting direct threats to human health. Through a series of communicative inversions achieved through public relations functions played by the media, think tanks, and universities as sites of knowledge production, the health-threatening elements of military interventions are rewritten into narratives that foreground military interventions as integral to democracy, justice, liberty, decontamination, containment, and promotion of well-being. The framing of terror and the articulations of discourses of terror erase from the discursive space the relationships of power and capital flow that simultaneously supply the instruments of violence to terror networks and state-sponsored military outfits. Moreover, these networks of military flow across the globe align local–global alliances among the transnational elite in flows of commodities, weapons, finances, and formal and informal labor. As I suggest in the next section, the networks of commodity flows intertwined with the intersecting relationships among the military also include flows in minerals, drugs, and oil.

A critical-cultural reading of health communication needs to examine the large-scale violent threats to health that are posed by wars and the consolidation of global power in the hands of the military. When wars are taken into account in regression equations mapping the many constructs that influence health, the strengths of the correlations accounted by technologies of violence are likely to be much larger than the health outcome correlations generated by eating five servings of fruits and vegetables and/or exercising. Yet much of the discourses of health communication are centered on interpretations of individual-level lifestyle factors that are likely to be dwarfed when compared with the negative health outcomes of war and violence. The health gains secured in a population by adopting exercising behavior are likely to be wiped out in one month of targeted bombing of a civilian population. What then are the interpretations and interpretive processes that render commonsense the violence constituted by war? The magnitudes of mortality produced by wars need to be accounted for in health communication theorizing, simultaneously attending to the communicative processes and interpretive frameworks that render acceptable such violent threats to human health and frame them as solutions of decontamination and containment. Scholars of health communication need to interrogate the interpretive processes and communicative inversions that render as common sense the logic of war as a neoliberal organizing framework of health promotion and disease containment.

Simultaneously, the complicity of academic knowledge production processes in supporting military interventions and in constituting neocolonialism needs to be closely interrogated, attending closely to the health consequences of these constructions. Academic research funded by the U.S. Department of Defense, for instance, continues to embody the colonial practice of knowledge production to achieve strategic military control. For instance, with the most recent U.S. invasions of Iraq and Afghanistan, the DoD has invested substantive resources in social scientific research, deploying anthropologists, political scientists, geographers, sociologists, psychologists, and communication scholars to decipher local cultures and to develop knowledge that would inform neocolonial interventions carried out by the United States, reflected in projects such as the human terrain systems (HTS) (HTS, n.d.).

The HTS work with academics in a variety of roles, including in roles as embedded social scientists, to decipher local cultures, to develop cultural maps, to decode cultural customs, and to deconstruct cultural narratives, all with the goal of informing more effective military practices in the "war on terror" (HTS, n.d.). The concept of culture, for instance, has configured in this body of work as a category to be deciphered and then to be incorporated into communicative strategies of war propaganda, psychological operations, public relations, and public opinion building (see, for instance, Corman, Hess & Justus, 2006). In the context of Operation Iraqi Freedom, the Center for Strategic Communication at Arizona State University funded by the DoD served as a space for knowledge production in establishing and reproducing U.S. hegemony. An introduction to one of the many white papers published by the center, titled *Credibility in the Global War on Terrorism*, argues (Corman et al., 2006):

> The perceived credibility of the United States government on the global stage has never been lower. This impedes its ability to fight, much less

> to win, the "war of ideas" that is so much a part of the global war on terrorism. Cultivating improved credibility is a long-term effort, but it stands to benefit from a large body of existing research. The concept of source credibility was developed by Aristotle in his classic text on effective communication, The Rhetoric. Formal efforts to manage U.S. credibility began in World War I. Modern social scientific research on the subject began during World War II and continues to the present day. More recent work has extended the concept to mass media and internet contexts.
>
> This body of research indicates that there are three key dimensions of credibility: trustworthiness, competence, and goodwill. These three dimensions are not empirical realities but perceptions that can be created, managed, and cultivated. This requires a coordinated approach to message design, delivery, and—most importantly—adaptation to the given audience and current media situation.

The role of academic research in communication is constructed as one of conducting analyses of persuasion strategies to identify ways of manipulating perceptions through a coordinated and strategic approach to message design. The articulation of a narrative framework is deployed toward developing effective persuasive strategies of manipulation for the U.S. military in its "war of ideas," framed within the ambits of the global war on terrorism. Academic knowledge in such a framework, conducted within the ambits of the military complex, works to further establish the hegemony of the military complex rather than interrogating the fundamental narratives circulated by the power structures, the materiality of these narratives, and the ways in which deceptive communication is deployed by the global power structures in achieving neocolonial control. Rather than critically interrogating the narrative of the "War on Terror," DoD-funded mainstream communication research works on strategies of establishing the hegemony of the narrative. Critical cultural interrogations of military and defense discourses attend to the communicative inequalities embodied in narratives such as the narrative of "War on Terror," attending to the ways in which such narratives perpetuate symbolic and material inequalities that threaten human health.

Military and Flow of Commodities, Minerals, and Wealth

In the global networks of power, the military is an integral player in the processes of wealth accumulation, playing an integral role in sustaining vastly unequal spaces of extraction and profit distribution. In mineral-rich areas of the globe, for instance, the lines between government and private militaries disappear as the military exerts power in enabling resource extraction, framed within the narrative of national development and geo-security (Harvey, 2005; Nordstrom, 2007). This network of military power also necessitates flows of arms, commodities, and a variety of products directed at serving the needs of the military. In her book *Global Outlaws*, Nordstrom observes:

> A large set of subsidiary businesses springs up to supply the lucrative industry of resource extraction. Soldiers, miners, middlemen, and concessionaries need mechanics, cooks, technical experts, shopkeepers, repair services, communications specialists, prostitutes. All of these people need food, cigarettes, alcohol, clothing, medicines, entertainment, tools, household of camping goods, transportation, and a host of related necessities and pleasures. (pp. 38–39)

The military is constituted amid the interconnected networks of commodity, labor, and capital flows, ensuring the flow of profits to the power elite and simultaneously itself creating new markets for products and commodities. Nordstrom further goes on to describe commodity networks as forming the lifelines of a country, mapping the military in the interflow of development, privatization and profiteering. She suggests (p. 42):

> Commodity networks are lifelines for a country. They anchor the complex interplay of economic development and profiteering: that kind of money can buy soldiers, sway politicians, even undermine governments; it can shape the course of development and of national policy.

It is worth noting here the intersections between the discourses of development and profiteering. Money, on one hand, buys and supports military networks and, on the other hand, is generated through the power of these military networks. The flow of money funding the military in local sites of control is tied to global networks of power.

In the context of Ogoniland in Nigeria, for instance, the transnational corporation Shell played a powerful role in supporting government-funded and privately financed military operations, suppressing dissent that challenged the oil-extracting profiteering objectives of Shell by voicing the health-threatening effects of Ogoni Dutch/Shell operations, the pollution and degradation of the environment, the exploitative extraction of profits, and the displacement of local communities from sources of livelihood by the oil extracting industry (Dutta, 2008, 2011; Pyagbara, 2007). Shell and the Nigerian military state worked in collusion in the use of violence to silence popular resistance, reflected in the hanging of the Nigerian activist

Ken Saro-Wiwa. On a similar note, large mining corporations in India work hand in hand with the state-funded military, deploying the narratives of development and security to thwart protests against the extractive processes (Padel & Das, 2010).

The local power of the military exerted in distant locales across the globe is intertwined with the global relationships of military power and military technologies that flow through development networks as well as through networks of legal and illegal trade. Money that flows across global borders in financing military operations is often tied to the agendas of global empire, the profiteering agendas of TNCs, and the collaborative relationships among the transnational elite. The United States, for instance, working through the funding and military aid structures of the Central Intelligence Agency (CIA), funded antidemocracy Contra rebel groups in Nicaragua, which in turn generated their funding through the illegal sale of drugs in African American communities in the United States, deploying profits from drug sales toward supporting the antidemocracy military interventions (Levine & Kavanau-Levine, 1993; Marcy, 2010; Villar, 2007; Webb, 1998). Such health-disruptive and health-threatening roles played by the military are whitewashed through an entire industry of communication experts working for large media houses and carrying out public relations functions (Cockburn, 1998; Villar, 2007).

Incarceration, Dissent, Racism, and Unequal Health

Across global sites of power, the proliferation of the military-industrial complex is accompanied by the rapid increase in the number of prisons globally, thus fundamentally affecting human health, life opportunities, and well-being across the life span (Massoglia, 2008). The neoliberal structures of governance are reproduced and protected through state-sponsored forms of violence that minimize opportunities of resistance, simultaneously privatizing prisons so that they become sites of labor extraction and profiteering (Hartnett, 2008). Take, for instance, the role of the police in controlling the possibilities of protest within the broader context of resisting the organizing structures of global finance. Protests in Occupy Wall Street were silenced through the deployment of armed police to evict protestors (Dutta, 2013a, 2013b). The global inequalities in distribution of wealth and the inequalities in health outcomes are reified and reproduced through the police-military structures, offering geosecurity as the justifying explanation for the erasure of democratic and participatory opportunities.

Moreover, dominant interpretations of race play key roles in shaping the role of the police as containing structures. For instance, immigrants of color at sites of protest in the United States are incarcerated, their protest being portrayed as terror, riot, and disruption rather than as democratic participation (Hartnett, 2008). The portrayals of race in articulations of civility and civil society underlie the neoliberal civilizing missions embodied in the various "wars on terror" carried out globally by the United States and its allies. Normative ideals of civility portrayed in mainstream discourses are intertwined with the civilizing missions of neocolonialism, embodying racist ideologies of power and control. For instance, the portrayals of Islam as the outside of civilization constitute neoliberal narratives of governmentality embodied in the global War on Terror. Torture and prisoner abuse are ironically routinized into the civilizing structures of the state, formulated on racist narratives of civility and civil society that mark the "other" as the outside of the civilization, thus rendering as common sense the uncivil use of violence and torture on the body of the other. Prisoner abuses in Guantanamo, Abu Ghraib, and across U.S. prisons globally are depicted discursively in the public relations functions of the mainstream press as deviance from the normative ideals of civility even as materially and symbolically these abuses are expressions of the underlying ideals of civility that mark the "other" as outside the realm of civilization and its civil processes.

Prisons emerge within this large-scale organizing of global structures as sites of controlling popular participation and protest, with the state playing an integral role in the resource consolidation processes and in deploying racist portrayals as justifications. I argue that the communicative inversions discussed throughout the book are tied to communicative erasures where spaces for protest, spaces for interrogation of the dominant ideologies, and spaces for articulations of alternatives are systematically silenced. The silencing of alternative rationalities is intrinsic to the reproduction of health-threatening global structures of power and wealth. Popular demands for social justice, accountability, and for redistribution of wealth are framed as threats to security and national development, often cast in the language of terrorism to justify the use of violence across the globe.

The police are increasingly deployed to control and manage neoliberal spaces, with public spaces and resources tied to market access, removing undesirable populations of color from these spaces. As urban redevelopment initiatives have emerged across urban centers, communities of color have been pushed out to the peripheries, marked as undesirable in the neoliberal aesthetic of the city as the cosmopolitan market. For instance, Samara (2010) depicts the ways in which private policing in urban spaces in South Africa reproduces the racial segregation of the apartheid era by tightly regulating the black urban poor through market-driven processes. Private security companies perform the policing function of tightly controlling global spaces to serve neoliberal agendas.

Prisons continue to serve as spaces for enacting racial disparities written into social organizing. In the United States, African Americans are significantly more likely to be incarcerated compared with Caucasians, embodying and reproducing race-specific health risks and risks to well-being (Goldberg, 2009). The structures of war are imbricated upon the depictions of spaces that are antithetical to neoliberal imaginations of whiteness as aberrations, subsequently justifying aggressive police and military responses. Sites of occupation secured through military force become sites of economic profiteering, often rhetorically leveraging the narrative of democracy as the façade for wealth extraction processes. Prisons, both publicly and privately funded, are reworked as public–private partnerships that are then sites of profiteering and exploitation of unpaid labor.

Surveillance and Health

The accumulation of wealth in the hands of the global elite operates on an instrumental logic of profiteering that is constituted within the overarching structure of neoliberal governmentality (Monahan, 2010). Global instruments of surveillance enabled through new technologies of power and control monitor global activism, sites of protest, and citizen participation in transformative politics. Private security corporations have been awarded contracts for surveillance, turning offline and online spaces under the gaze of the panopticon (Monahan, 2010). Projects of surveillance in universities are funded by the global power structures to gather intelligent information on social change processes, to map such information, and to use such information in planning and response. Global organizations such as the National Security Agency (NSA) carry out surveillance and monitoring functions that gather intelligence and feed data to transnational decision-making structures. Surveillance of social and mobile media feed into these global structures of power and control.

Deviants, marked as abnormal manifestations and therefore as threats to the neoliberal order, are kept under instruments of surveillance (Dutta, 2013b). Resources directed at public welfare are shifted into resources for surveillance and management. Rather than offer social and public health support programs for the underserved, neoliberal reforms develop work programs for extracting labor and simultaneously create an array of surveillance technologies for watching over the deviant workers. Technologies of surveillance such as cameras foster spaces for extracting labor.

Health and disease, constructed in the language of biosecurity, are positioned within these structures of surveillance, securing access to health data and scanning such data to map out patterns of disease (Teutsch & Churchill,

2000). Health data become subjects of examination and prediction, being analyzed by security teams looking for patterns, anomalies, and threats. Biological samples and specimens are closely examined with an emphasis on developing timely response strategies. The proliferation of discourses of privacy is constituted amid penetrating structures of examination that dig deep into the body and the cellular structures to decipher threats. The next section specifically attends to the languages and meanings of aggression and control that constitute the neoliberal security apparatus.

Language, Aggression, and Control

In this section, we specifically attend to the ways in which the dominant interpretations and meanings within neoliberal structures foreground the framework of security, connecting disease to security and necessitating security responses to health needs. We also attend to the implications of this overarching security framework in approaching health and disease.

Security, Economics, and Disease

Disease outbreaks are framed as threats to security and economics, continuing to reify the colonial logics of disease response, albeit framed in the language of the interconnected links between local, national, and global economies. The anthrax attacks in the backdrop of 9/11 fostered openings for the narrative of biosecurity, with large-scale mobilization of resources in the United States toward biosecurity response, connecting the realm of the bio with the neoliberal structures of security, and shaping science within the structure of global geosecurity. The war metaphor played a key role in the response of the Singapore government to SARS, amplifying specific sense of crisis vulnerabilities among citizens to chart out military responses to the disease (Ibrahim, 2007). The security frame was thus also intrinsically tied to the nation-building frame, appealing to narratives of moral responsibility, patriotism, and economic progress to build opinion and action.

In the depiction of SARS, the WHO report issued in 2003 states:

> At this moment, public health authorities, doctors, nurses, scientists, and laboratory staff around the world are struggling to cope with SARS at a time when some hope remains that the disease might still be contained. Economists and market analysts are simultaneously struggling to calculate the present and future costs, initially estimated at US$30 billion in the Far East alone. Public panic is widespread, some

> government officials have lost their jobs, and social stability has been jeopardized in some of the hardest hit areas.

Note the intersections of economics, market analysis, and social stability in the depiction of SARS. Here, the economic costs are projected by WHO globally, with specific references to the economic costs to the Far East alone. Teams of market analysts and economists occupy the discursive sphere, deployed to calculate the costs of disease threats. The uncertainty around SARS is played out in the uncertainty of economic modeling, directed at mapping out the amount of economic loss that has been caused by SARS. Collaborative hubs and spaces for shared research within and between nation-states were constituted under the structure of security.

Similarly, the discursive climate around 9/11 was shaped in the language of security, simultaneously creating a new global market around the surveillance and management of threats. For instance, consider the emergence of a new market of bio-detection technologies such as microchips for detecting biohazards as mechanisms for ensuring the security of those who sit in positions of power. The anthrax attacks, accompanied by the 9/11 attacks fostered the climate for U.S. investments into biosecurity under the structure of homeland security and emergency preparedness. The language of biosecurity offers a taxonomy for disease response where the scientific research into biological threats is framed within military and security structures, and the corresponding crisis responses and strategies are formulated within the organizing structure of the military (Koblentz, 2010).

Military Metaphor

One of the core elements of the military deployed toward AIDS relief within the ambits of PEPFAR is the U.S. Military HIV Research Program (MHRP). The function of the MHRP is to conduct HIV research within the purview of the military. The role of health-related knowledge production to serve the goals of the military becomes evident in the many documents and publications of the MHRP. Consider, for instance, the following articulation on the occasion of World Malaria Day on April 25, 2014 (www.hivresearch.org/news.php?NewsID=293) in a press release titled "How the Military Is Engaged in the Battle against Malaria":

> For the U.S. military, as far back as 1775, George Washington had to expend his very limited monetary resources to purchase quinine for the treatment of malaria in the Revolutionary Army. During the Civil War, 50 percent of Caucasian troops and a staggering 80 percent

> of African-American troops contracted malaria annually. Conflicts within the last century continue to highlight the threat of malaria to our troops with World War II, Vietnam, and even recently in Afghanistan. Malaria can have a significant operational impact: in 2003 a military peacekeeping operation in Liberia failed due to 80 cases of malaria in 220 Marines within the first few weeks of the mission.

Note the title of the message that constructs the role of the military in fighting the battle against disease. The military metaphor works literally to deploy military functions toward fighting disease.

Tracing the history of treatment of malaria in the Revolutionary Army, the depiction presents the role of disease prevention to protecting the military troops. For instance, the depiction of the percent of troops that contracted malaria during the Civil War communicates the threat posed by malaria to the war mission. Disease is depicted as an aggressor that threatens the aggressive agendas of the military. Recent examples of the threat of malaria to troops in Afghanistan and Liberia are presented to suggest that failure in operations may result from the threats posed by health. Once again, the threats posed by disease add to the threats to be conquered by the military.

The military metaphor is tied to the narrative of economic development and growth. Consider further: "Despite many progress in diseases prevention and treatment over the last several decades, malaria continues to threaten the lives of millions of children and adults and hamper economic development." Malaria as a threat connects human health to the neoliberal logic of economic development and growth. The military is seen as a resource for protecting the agendas of economic development. On a similar note, the release documents the amount of economic resources that have historically been spent on fighting malaria. References are made to the resources and expenditures.

Moreover, the threats to military operations are connected with broader threats to the geosecurity of the global elite posed by poverty. Poverty is thus seen as a threat that needs to be managed through military strategy rather than being interpreted as a product of the very structures of neoliberalism that constitute global inequalities and the large-scale impoverishment of the poor. By situating the structural contexts of health in the background and by connecting health to military interventions, the neoliberal framework of governance necessitates military interventions as responses to problems of global health. Specifically relevant are the constructions of health as threats that call for the deployment of military technologies as tools for disciplining. For instance, the war narrative emerged as a dominant thread in global responses to SARS across spaces of economic production. Similarly, in response to the recent outbreaks of Ebola in parts of West Africa, including Sierra Leone and Liberia, the United States deployed military forces as strategic responses to the health crisis (Berman, 2014). The military metaphor draws upon the narrative of war to justify the uses of force and violence as tools of disciplining that are required to contain threats to health, embodied in quarantine measures that limit access to health services, care, and adequate health supplies among the target populations. Moreover, the presence of the military as a solution consolidates greater power in the hands of the military as an organizational structure that serves the geostrategic and economic interests of the power elite.

Vulnerabilities and Anxieties

Inherent to epidemics in a globalized world is the sense of embodied vulnerability, manifesting the anxieties rooted in one's sense of their place in an increasingly interconnected world, networked through movements of materials, resources, and labor (Aaltola, 2012; Everts, 2013). These anxieties and vulnerabilities are distributed in uneven and unequal terrains of power and profits. Distribution of wealth plays a pivotal role in shaping the nature and structure of surveillance, security, and crisis response programs, pointing to the structural features of neoliberalism and generating response measures that privilege those with economic access. Yet these structural features of global disease vulnerabilities, constituted amid large-scale global inequalities, displacements, climate change patterns, and patterns of resource accumulation, are overshadowed by individualized models of anxieties that emphasize individual responsibility, ownership, and participation in the market. Putting forth a managerial framework, crisis response is seen as a mechanism for mapping out, responding to, and evaluating these vulnerabilities, feeding into an entire industry of communication and management experts that are organized to keep the system intact and return it to a state of normalcy through an emphasis on the individual consumer.

Responses framed as security and crisis response strategies reify the structures of inequalities that constitute health vulnerabilities. Anxieties thus are located in the realm of the individual and solutions are specifically channeled toward addressing the psycho-affective elements of anxiety directed at promoting specific behavioral responses. Neoliberal governmentality offers private–public militarized solutions as responses to the anxieties, with solutions emphasizing the development of new technologies of surveillance, coordination, management, and crisis response (Caballero, 2005; Caballero-Anthony, 2006). Communication is conceived of as technologies of information gathering, information filtering, information dissemination, coordination, strategy, and persuasion, with the goal of gathering relevant information to shape response strategies and then disseminate these strategies through effective channels. The quality of communication strategies is measured in frameworks of criteria such as resilience, fidelity, timeliness, and efficiency.

Disease as Bioterror

A dominant trope that circulates in mainstream discourses of emerging and infectious disease is the trope of bioterror, suggesting terrorist threats that need to be controlled through appropriate military intelligence gathering and intervention. Consider the following statement issued by George W. Bush in June 2002, "Bioterrorism is a real threat to our country. It's a threat to every nation that loves freedom. Terrorist groups seek biological weapons; we know some rogue states already have them. . . . It's important that we confront these real threats to our country and prepare for future emergencies." This narrative identifies the source of terror as outside the structures of the mainstream power configurations, threatening to disrupt the economic, political, and social stability of these structures. The global free market economy is framed as the love for freedom, and bioterror threats are articulated as disruptions to this global free market. Yet what remains erased from the discursive space is the origin of much of biological weapons from within the military establishment structures of dominant nation-states in the global North within the context of the world wars and the Cold War (Croddy, Hart & Perez-Armendariz, 2002). Even as the source of threat is cast on terrorists from elsewhere, the large-scale military investments in biowarfare are hidden from the discursive space.

The deployment of the bioterror narrative works to situate disease response within the ambits of military surveillance and response.

> Efforts to improve global capacity to address microbial threats should be coordinated with key international agencies such as the World Health Organization (WHO) and based in the appropriate U.S. federal agencies (e.g., the Centers for Disease Control and Prevention [CDC], the Department of Defense [DoD], the National Institutes of Health [NIH], the Agency for International Development [USAID], the Department of Agriculture [USDA], with active communication and coordination among these agencies and in collaboration with private organizations and foundations. Investments should take the form of financial and technical assistance, operational research, enhanced surveillance, and efforts to share both knowledge and best public health practices across national boundaries. (Smolinski, Hamburg & Lederberg, 2003, p. 151)

In the above depiction, the portrayal of microbial threats works toward mobilizing the coordinated response integrating the military (DoD) with public health, development, and agriculture. The deployment of the bioterror narrative serves as the basis for surveillance, the development of response infrastructures, and integration of efforts across global boundaries. Intelligence gathering and monitoring is coupled with effective prevention and protection, surveillance, and response and recovery.

The neoliberal organizing of health deploys the narrative of bioterror to shape and circulate anxieties around infectious diseases, thus offering the bases for the development of military solutions in order to secure boundaries against the free flow of disease in a global marketplace that is predicated on the free flow of capital, labor, goods, and markets. In this sense, the military emerges as an instrument of disciplining the flow of labor and commodities in order to ensure the hegemony of neoliberal governance, balancing between the competing needs of globalization. Whereas on one hand the neoliberal construction of infectious diseases captures the continuity with colonial depictions that connect infectious disease with questions of geosecurity and economic development in the context of the empire, on the other hand, neoliberal framing of emerging infectious diseases maps out a global structure of networks of surveillance, information dissemination, prevention, and control to effectively manage the movement of disease across the open borders that are necessary for the free market (King, 2002). Coordination, collaboration, and networking emerge as key strategies for fighting the threats of bioterrorism.

Racist Depictions

The deployment of policies to demarcate, quarantine, discipline, and manage spaces is constituted around constructions of threats to global geosecurity (King, 2002; Sastry & Dutta, 2012). These constructions often depict the body of the "other" as a threat, drawing upon colonial notions of pollution to justify the implementation of policies of separation and quarantine, marking out bodies to be kept out of neoliberal spheres (Keil & Ali, 2008). The depictions of race are intertwined with depictions of class, with disproportionate emphases on controlling the flow of the underclasses across global borders, paradoxically situated amid the fundamental role played by these underclasses in supplying underpaid labor to global economies. Notions of purity that are intrinsically connected to dominant ideas of race are utilized as strategies for categorization and mapping within multicultural spaces of neoliberal governance (Sastry & Dutta, 2012). The policing and mapping of urban spaces depict the fissures in the multicultural narratives of neoliberalism, justifying policies of separation on the basis of markers of purity and impurity.

Prevailing perceptions of class intersect with perceptions of race in the articulation and implementation of security policies. For instance, in global spaces of management of emerging disease, migrant workers, essential to the global economy as sources of cheap and exploited labor, are turned into bodies to be managed. In the case of Singapore's response to SARS, all foreign workers who came to Singapore to work as construction workers had to go through a fourteen-day quarantine at an isolated location whereas foreign professionals working in Singapore as well as Singaporeans who had visited SARS-affected countries were asked to voluntarily quarantine themselves for ten days (Teo, Yeoh & Ong, 2005). The design and implementation of the quarantine policies depicting the differential treatment of foreign construction workers subjected to the fourteen-day mandatory quarantine vis-à-vis the foreign professionals subjected to a voluntary ten-day quarantine depict the role of class as an organizing frame for policy implementation in the context of managing migrant worker populations.

Global pandemics make evident the uneven relationships of power between the global North and the global South. The experiences of anxiety in the global North about contamination from the unruly and polluted global South form the bases for controls on global movements, especially movements originating from the poorer sectors of the global South. A variety of strategies of containment are designed and implemented, often depicting the uneven flows of power. Uneven quarantine policies and policies of segregation are examples of the interplay of race in global military networks of power and control. Racist depictions of cultural practices in China, for instance, were integral to global military responses to the SARS pandemic. The power of the military in organizing and disciplining bodies, in examining bodies by penetrating them, and in disciplining the flow of bodies is intertwined with dominant ideas and frames of race and purity of the body (Larson, Nerlich & Wallis, 2005). Notions of contamination depicting colonial logics are integral to the practices of segregation that are carried out through the deployment of the military (Chiang & Duann, 2007). Similarly, the military is also a crucial player in the distribution of resources in response to crises, working to support the security of dominant power structures as the primary agenda.

Strategies of Neoliberal Governance

The role of communication is integral to the securitization of health, with communicative functions being played out in the form of uncertainty management and information gathering, prevention and behavior change, and crisis response and recovery. In this section, we specifically examine these functions of communication within the broader structures of biodefense and biosecurity.

Managing Uncertainty and Knowledge

The control of disease outbreak is predicated upon the effective management of uncertainty through the production of knowledge. Given the very uncertainty produced around emerging disease and the limited existing knowledge in coping with the rapid spread of the disease, neoliberal governmentality emphasizes the effective management of uncertainty through the paradoxical foci on accelerated knowledge production, on one hand, and the simultaneous management of crises response constituted around the uncertainty produced by the very nature of the disease, on the other hand. Research and development investments are poured into developing knowledge and intelligence structures directed at predicting the next outbreak and the appropriate strategies for containing the outbreak on a global scale. Such monolithic emphases on surveillance mechanisms ignore the very nature of emerging infectious diseases, grounded in uncertainties in the nature of knowledge, nature of knowledge claims, and the processes of production of these knowledge claims.

The depictions of disease around the inherent tensions between certainty and uncertainty call for information-gathering strategies that would unmask the face of the disease. Consider the following depiction of SARS in the WHO (2003) report on SARS, under the subtitle "Unmasking a New Disease":

> WHO maintains its position that SARS can and must be contained—pushed back out of its new human host. One by one, the many puzzling features of this new disease are being unmasked. One by one, the most severe outbreaks in the initial waves of infection are being brought under control. Recommended measures—case detection, isolation and infection control, and contact tracing and follow-up surveillance—are working. With this reassurance, the image of populations masked because of fear, the public face of SARS, can now begin to fade. (p. 41)

The fundamental ontological uncertainty rooted in the very nature of SARS is reflected in the depiction of the puzzling features of the disease. The function of the network of global experts then is constituted around unmasking the puzzle, in figuring out the key elements of the puzzle, and in developing adequate strategies for controlling the uncertainty. The specific steps of case detection, isolation, infection control, contact tracing, and surveillance are set up as global mechanisms of collaborations within the networks of response. The affect rooted in the uncertainties of the disease and its threats of movement across boundaries is dealt with through the deployment of effective management strategies.

The anxieties that are constituted around the uncertainties that lie fundamental to the unknown nature of emerging infectious diseases call for effective and efficient uncertainty management. Management of uncertainty is constituted around knowing the exact roots of the disease, identifying and locating the point of origin of the disease, identifying the points of contact and the infection hot spots, effectively quarantining these hot spots, and managing public behavior with a limited level of knowledge. At different stages of the pandemic, expert teams work on the various aspects of identifying and locating disease flows, constituted amid the very uncertainties produced by the rapid global flows of material and labor in a globalized world. The uncertainty around emerging infectious diseases also then feeds into an embodied sense of vulnerability in an interconnected world, manifest in the rapid flow of goods, services, and people across borders. The heightened sense of vulnerability which I argue is itself constituted by global flows is tied to the disproportionate anxieties that are circulated.

Intelligence Gathering

Intelligence gathering about potential disease threats across global spaces has emerged as a key function of neoliberal governance, bringing health under the umbrella of military surveillance, often packaged in the form of biodefense and fighting bioterrorism through intelligent responses. Information gathering takes center stage in strategic response functions (Kreps et al., 2005). Effective intelligence gathering in this model gathers information about potential threats and alerts the system about likely outbreaks before they take the shape of outbreaks. Monitoring media reports, new media, and social media, for instance, emerges as a strategy for identifying potential biological threats early on, mapping diffusion and dissemination patterns through analyses and predicting appropriate response strategies. Neoliberal governmentality invests in early warning systems in order to alert global structures of power about potential risks so that these risks can be quickly managed. Inherent in the notion of intelligence gathering is the notion of controlling uncertainty in spite of the very uncertain, unpredictable, and fluid nature of disease outbreaks.

The connection between health and terror serves as a mechanism for deploying global structures of surveillance under the auspices of the military. Note, for instance, the following depiction of prevention of biological threats by Kreps et al. (2005, p. 355):

> Intelligence gathering activities involve actively seeking regular updates from extensive networks of informants and organizational contacts to

> uncover threatening plans and activities. Biohazard intelligence is also gathered through close (and often unobtrusive) surveillance of group activities and environmental conditions that might identify risk factors and indicators, including monitoring communications among terrorist groups, tracking any unauthorized or suspicious access to contagious substances, and identifying epidemiologic evidence of biological contagion and disease from around the world.

Gathering adequate and effective information about the disease are seen as critical communication elements in disease response. Surveillance functions are seen as critical components in detecting potential threats and in developing adequate response strategies. Intelligence in this sense is directed at gathering information ahead of time in order to prevent outbreak.

Yet the very nature of disease outbreaks points toward the limits of the intelligence gathering mechanisms. Consider, for instance, the WHO (2003, p. 1) report on SARS that dances between the depictions of uncertainty and certainty:

> SARS is the first severe and readily transmissible new disease to emerge in the 21st century. Though much about the disease remains poorly understood and frankly puzzling, SARS has shown a clear capacity for spread along the routes of international air travel. At present, the outbreaks of greatest concern are concentrated in transportation hubs or spreading in densely populated areas. WHO regards every country with an international airport, or bordering an area having recent local transmission, as at potential risk of an outbreak.

Note here the depiction of the poor and incomplete nature of current level of understanding of the SARS puzzle amid the sense of certainty that is then offered through depiction of specific information on the routes of transmission of SARS. Given the nature of the uncertainty, the intelligence that is generated by WHO in this case points to the obvious and the generic, suggesting that every country with an international airport is at potential risk of an outbreak.

Networks of Information

The effective gathering of relevant and precise information is coupled with the development of robust networks for information flow and information sharing. The language of diffusion offers an interpretive frame for studying networks of information flow and for developing explanatory and predictive models for mapping disease spread. Teams of scientific experts collaborate with military and management personnel to build network infrastructures for crisis response. An array of pundits, public relations professionals, crisis response professionals, and media professionals come together in framing the issue, highlighting specific interpretations, and in disseminating specific forms of information around the dominant issue frames. The sense of urgency and crisis is integral to the development of rapid response teams for effective management of the crisis (Everts, 2013). Health organizations such as the U.S. Centers for Disease Control and Prevention (CDC) become sites for developing issue frames and information packages that are then disseminated through broader networks that include the media, military, and social networks on emerging and new media (Everts, 2013).

Crisis Communication

Framing pandemics as biological threats, the zeitgeist of communication interventions emphasize the development of appropriate communication strategies to induce quick behavior change (such as hand washing), control fears and anxieties, direct movement of people across spaces, and provide information on available prevention, treatment, and response information (Slezak et al., 2003). Kreps et al. (2005), for instance, note the vital role of media relations in coordinating information dissemination functions to achieve fidelity in the information that is put out by state agencies and other allied actors. The organizing framework of risk and crisis communication is seen as laying out communication strategies for handling risks and for effectively communicating about them with members of the public as well as various stakeholder groups (Chitnis, 2012).

The languages of emergency preparedness and disease responsiveness shape the overarching structure for defining the constructions of global public health (see Garrett, 1996). Resources are invested into simulations and drills for developing, fine-tuning, and testing crisis response strategies. Take, for instance, the mainstream discourses around the avian flu and the corresponding crises response strategies. The deployment of crisis response strategies is focused on promoting specific behavioral responses, constituted amid limited understanding of these behavioral responses, their effectiveness and side effects, the costs involved, and the broader context of risks.

Disease Control as a Management Function

One of the features of neoliberal governance is the deployment of managerial language in the containment of flow of people and goods across the globe. This is a critical challenge of neoliberal governance, given the dependence of global neoliberal hegemony on the mobility and flexibility of labor and capital. Given the limited nature of knowledge that is often available about a particular disease when it breaks out, the strategies of response often resort to the colonial strategies of isolation and quarantine, reformulated within a narrative of effective management. Hospital and government management strategies are identified in a framework of best practices that offer the recipe for action.

Let's refer to a WHO (2006) report on SARS. The report notes (p. 246):

> In a globalized world, where people and products travel vast distances virtually in an instant, threats to health, whether real or imagined, can be economically disastrous. The economic devastation wreaked by SARS is well documented. Billions of dollars were lost by countries ill prepared for such losses, particularly in the tourism, hospitality, and transport industries. A clearly reasoned, well-planned, and effectively managed and publicized response to such threats is important in mitigating the damage to the economy, and to public confidence in government.

Effective disease management is seen as integral to achieving public trust in government, confidence in government, and in mitigating threats to the economy. The overarching framework of securing the economy resonates throughout the document, depicting the neoliberal interpretive frame of economics-driven intervention management.

Terms such as *super-spreader*, *carrier*, and *recipient* are circulated in disease control and management frameworks as entry points for identifying and isolating the sources of the disease and for containing further spread (Aaltola, 2012). References to "index cases" and "super-spreader events" offer ontological categories for interpreting infectious disease diffusion patterns and for intervening into these patterns effectively, rapidly, and efficiently. Models of network structures and network relationships are mapped out as strategies of containment. Programs of training of health workers, managers, media and public relations experts, providers, and government officials are constructed within a management framework, with the police and military playing key roles in the management response structures. Moreover, both popular and news media frames pick up and circulate the narrative of disease management as an overarching framework.

Disease Control as Disciplining

Given the emphasis on containment, disciplining the movement of human bodies emerges as a predominant trope in neoliberal disease management. In response to the outbreak of SARS, disease response played out in the deployment of appropriate strategies for controlling movement and for controlling the flow of the disease, often carrying out security and military responses in order to contain the flow of the disease. Consider the following excerpt from the WHO (2003, p. 2) report:

> In Hong Kong, an electronic tracking system developed by the police force for use in criminal investigations has been adapted for contact tracing and monitoring of compliance with quarantine. In Singapore, military forces have been deployed to assist in contact tracing and to enforce quarantines that have halted the normal lives of thousands of people. No visitors are allowed at any public hospital.

Containment as a disciplining strategy renders as common sense the intervention by the military. Health is framed as a threat that needs to be managed by controlling power over populations through the instruments of the military, silencing the healing possibilities of health. The military is put forth in a management framework, where the management of the disease is itself a military function that needs to be streamlined in the managerial structure of effectiveness and efficiency.

Conclusion

In this chapter, we paid close attention to the global discourses of geosecurity, freedom, and economic growth that play pivotal roles in the securitization of disease. As the security framework emerges as the governing principle for guiding and managing public–private partnerships directed at informing, educating, and persuading the individual target, questions of economic inequalities and disparities in distribution of resources remain erased from the discursive space. The gaps in global distribution of health resources and the role of neoliberal interventions in contributing to the widening of these gaps remain absent from an overarching framework of geosecurity. The privileging of the economic context and costs of a disease fundamentally contributes to inequitable priorities, with emphasis placed on serving the health needs of those segments of the population that are economically profitable and provide viable markets for health solutions. Under the neoliberal model, fundamental health needs of poor and underserved populations are often erased from the discursive space while increasing investments in technologies of security and response are directed toward serving the needs of the transnational elite. Moreover, the centrality of the market logic channels large-scale public research funding into developing health solutions, which are subsequently privatized and sold through the market.

The interplay of race and social class draw attention to the inequalities of health that continue to be reproduced by an overarching framework of geosecurity tied to protecting economic interests. As recently observed in the context of Ebola, the networks of flow of global disease response embody racist tropes that differentially value human life, with the absence of public health infrastructures to meet the needs of the poor underclasses across the globe. With the hegemony of the public–private framework as the solution pushed by the IFIs, global, national, and public health infrastructures have been weakened, thus unable to respond adequately to Ebola. The absence of local capacities in providing basic care is manifest in the absence of providers, medical supplies, and adequate response systems. Instead, the reframing of disease in military terms privileges geosecurity with an emphasis on quarantine and segregation. Whether it is the communities in Sierra Leone or the African American communities in New Orleans, the weakening of public infrastructures to support the poor bring forth the fault lines of neoliberalism. Yet these fault lines remain erased from discursive spaces of global disease surveillance and management that emphasize new technologies of surveillance and crises response through market mechanisms and through military responses (Farmer, 2001). The reframing of global health in the language of security fundamentally weakens the infrastructures of public health that are intrinsic to promoting equitable, just, and accessible health environments and health care.

CHAPTER SEVEN

COMMUNICATION TECHNOLOGIES AND HEALTH

In Chapter Seven, attention will be paid to the global emergence of technology as a framework for the delivery of health. The technological discourse of health is a key tenet of the free market rationality, shaping health as a technological solution, and therefore connecting health to the logics of commoditization in the market, shaping solutions to global health inequalities as mediatized through communication technologies. Technological determinism refers to the prevailing interpretation of technology as the magic bullet the dissemination of which will produce planned effects in targeted populations, and has been at the heart of the modernist framework of development that later morphed into the neoliberal framework of global health governance. The hegemonic framing of technology as an innovation forms the basis of the widely adopted diffusion of innovations theory that forms the bulwark of much communication scholarship originating from the early conceptualizations of development communication. Terms such as *new media*, *cyber-revolution*, and *information revolution* are put forth in order to frame technology as the solution to problems of health, and in order to predict the next health revolution. The pervasive global presence of neoliberal health organizing has seen the accelerated adoption of health technologies as the predominant and often the exclusive solutions to problems of global health, simultaneously obfuscating the structural inequities that are often produced by communicative processes and processes of material production brought about by these technologies, minimizing the threats to health posed by technologies, and erasing the narratives of job loss, unemployment, exploitation, and weakened organizing capacity of labor within the broader context of new technologies (Guvenen, 2013; Harris et al., 2013).

Building technological infrastructures is seen as a way for building community capacity in disenfranchised communities, complemented by message tailoring and message targeting strategies directed at targeted populations, selected through specific measures of risk (Harris et al., 2013). Technologies of measurement shape technologies of message design delivered through new and innovative design technologies. Increasingly, the emphasis is on new cycles of innovation, investing in new innovations that would create more sophisticated technologies, more sophisticated methods of delivery, and more sophisticated methods of message development. These targeted populations are described as underserved populations, and technologically mediated interventions are directed at them with the goal of addressing inequities of access and cultural barriers to health and well-being. Erased from the discursive space are articulations of the distribution of resources and the broader structural configurations that constitute health. Also erased from a predominantly technologically deterministic framework are considerations of alternative rationalities of health that challenge the reductionist logics of biomedical technologies, the adverse health impacts of these technologies, and the negative health outcomes associated with the uncritical adoption of a technological hegemony. Also erased are the cultural meanings constituted around these technologies that are pushed as solutions to health in target communities. The accelerated push for the "newer and better" is often accompanied by the erasure of democratic spaces for the discussion of the underlying science, the potential implications of the science, the associated costs and questions of affordability, and the possibilities of adverse side effects. Conflicts of interest in the processes of the production of the innovation are written in as normalized features of the framework of development, as necessities that facilitate innovation, thus backgrounding opportunities for authentic debate based on data and evidence. Processes of research and development, design, production, implementation, dissemination, and evaluation of these technologies are increasingly rendered opaque, inaccessible to spaces of public discourse and public participation.

Moreover, the technologically mediated framework of global organizing has formed the basis of global shifts in movements of capital, labor, and resources, with technology playing a key role in the offshoring of jobs, the automation of jobs, the financialization of capital, the diffusion of innovations to new markets, and the surveillance of labor, markets, and resources. Technology operates on the logic of maximizing the efficiency and productivity of systems, as well as closely monitoring systems to ensure the greatest profits for innovators, entrepreneurs, and TNCs transacting in these technologies. All of this has been accomplished through the organizing structure of the narrative of development, with technology being equated with development, economic growth, and as solutions to poverty and inequality. The networks of financial capital flow through communication technologies; information is circulated and transactions are made on these technologically mediated platforms. Technological innovations thus have been integral to neoliberal processes of resource consolidation, playing central roles in the consolidation of power in the hands of the global elite and in the global ascendance of the managerial class.

This chapter works through the traces of discourse that depict the intersections of technology, expertise, the market logic, and the ways in which these intersections work together toward the consolidation of resources in the hands of the global elite. We begin by looking at mainstream frameworks of organizing technology in global structures, situating these frameworks in the context of communicative processes and the flow of communication. We then interrogate the health correlates of a techno-deterministic framework, wrapping up the chapter with a critical interrogation of the technologies of health.

Mainstream Framework of Technology

In the mainstream framework, technology is treated as an innovation in the processes of development and growth, and this emphasis on bringing about transformations in health and development forms the roots of development communication. Where development in the form of modernization principles takes place in the shape of a linear trajectory, technology is seen as a positive good that will bring about social change in primitive populations in the pathway of development. Underdeveloped or undeveloped economies therefore, it is believed, will move into stages of development through the adoption of new technologies. Earliest communication interventions were driven by the agenda of disseminating technologies such as agricultural technologies and population control as strategies for bringing about modernization in targeted societies conceived as primitive or lacking in the metrics of development.

The essence of this dichotomization between the primitive and the modern is witnessed in Everett Rogers' (1974, 1983, 1995, 2003) diffusion of innovations framework, the dominant theoretical framework of development communication that captures the technology-centered thinking. In recalling his early interest in diffusion of innovations, Rogers shares the story of his farmer family and neighbors in rural Iowa, asking the basis of differentiation between the farmers that adopted new agricultural innovations and the farmers that stuck to age old methods, depicting the powerful role of agricultural technologies in the Cold War development communication discourse. This bias toward technology is well captured in the description of Rogers' early interest in innovations described by Singhal and Deering (2006, p. 17):

> Back at his farm, Ev observed that his father loved electro-mechanical farm innovations; but was resistant to biological-chemical innovations. For instance, Ev's father resisted adopting the new hybrid seed

> corn, even though it yielded 25 percent more crop, and was resistant to drought. However, during the Iowa drought of 1936, while the hybrid seed corn stood tall on the neighbors' farm, the crop on the Rogers' farm wilted. Ev's father was finally convinced. It took him eight years to make up his mind. These questions about innovation diffusion, including the strong resistances, and how they could be overcome, formed the core of Ev's graduate work.

Inherent then in the role of communication as conceived within this dominant framework is the defining role of technology as an all-encapsulating solution, as well as a resource for disseminating innovations in target communities. The technology itself is taken for granted as the solution within the interpretive frame, with communication narrowly being conceived as strategies of dissemination. With an emphasis on delving into the strategies of persuasion, the positivistic framing of technology leaves intact the interpretive frames around the technology. The contestations, community voices, and critical interrogations of technologies as instruments of power remain erased from discursive spaces. The mainstream structure of communication is deeply intertwined with the Western/white liberal fetish with technology as the modern solution to health and development, replicating the Cold War frame that envisioned technology as an instrument in the growth process that would recruit target countries in the Third World into the Western/white liberal framework of capitalism and simultaneously resist the communist movements that were growing across the newly independent colonies. Fundamental questions of communication that highlight interpretation, meaning, and discourse are erased from the discursive spaces of mainstream communication research, theorizing, and practice. The technology bias thus plays out in the uncritical adoption of technological innovations as solutions of health and well-being, leaving unquestioned issues of adverse effects, side effects, societal-level impacts, and so on.

In other words, the role of communication is in disseminating the technology, and communication research is guided by the quest for new technologies, processes, and strategies for disseminating the technologies. The mainstream framework of communication has historically been constituted around the search for communication technologies for disseminating a variety of technologies of modernity such as population control and its later version of family planning (see Chapter Two), agricultural biotechnology (see Chapter Three), free market economy, democracy, civil society, and so forth. In this framework, communication has been traditionally conceived of as a positive resource is the form of technology. The dissemination of the communication technology is taken for granted as a positive outcome, disconnected from empirical evidence regarding the outcomes of the technology, without the consideration of broader social-political-economic-cultural contexts, and without taking into account the patterns of ownership of the technology. Also erased are questions of profiteering and market economics that are tied to the dissemination of these technologies.

This dichotomy between pre- and post-states and the role of technology in enabling the transformation from one state to another forms the basis of contemporary neoliberal governance, albeit at an accelerated pace, and achieved through the consolidation of technology in the hands of private capital. For instance, in referring to technology as a harbinger of freedom, Lin (2007) draws upon the articulations of Poole (1982) to suggest that new communication technologies are likely to challenge totalitarian state systems. On a similar note, Lin (2007) suggests the positive role of technology in the context of newly emerging democracies in the former communist bloc countries. Similarly, in contemporary frameworks discussing the role of technology in the context of social change processes in the Arab Spring, techno-deterministic understandings of technology put forth the role of technology as a catalyst for citizen participation, engagement, and democratic transition. Citizenship, democracy, and civil society become enabled through the ownership of private technologies. In addition, the creation of innovations such as democracy and civil societies is intertwined with the creation of markets for commoditized technologies such as computers, internet, and social media such as Facebook and Twitter.

Technology thus is conceived of as an equalizer, with the underlying notion that creating access to technology will equalize broader structural forms of inaccess. Here, access to technology is seen as an individual level enabler, creating access for the individual and her/his family to a wide range of resources through the introduction of the technology. Fundamentally, technology is conceptualized as the solution to lack of access to a variety of basic resources such as food, health, and shelter. If an individual, household, or community is connected with the basic elements of technology, the technology can serve as the gateway for securing access to these basic resources. Communication programs therefore are built around the notion of building communication infrastructures across global communities accompanied by the development of communication training programs for community members. Those sectors of the population are defined as disenfranchised or underserved that have no or limited access to technology resources. Technology becomes a tool for empowering marginalized community members.

Under the neoliberal regime of global social change processes, technology is foregrounded as the solution to the large-scale inequalities that have been generated by a technology-centered, expert-driven model of resource consolidation. That technology is integral to the processes of automation, to the flexible movement of labor, and to the development of global networks of offshore manufacturing and resource extraction that constitute the landscape of inequalities remains erased from the discursive space that puts forth technology as the solutions to these symptoms of inequalities. Instead, the framing of new communication technologies as instruments for addressing global health challenges fosters new markets for start-ups, entrepreneurs, and commercial ventures. Inequalities can be apparently addressed through new "apps" and "technological interfaces," recreating new markets for the very technological commodities that underlie large-scale patterns of global inequalities. Erased from the mainstream framework of technology are discussions of the role of technologies in shaping the global textures of inequalities, poverty, health inequality, weakening of public health, and lack of access to basic infrastructures of public health in the global South. Also erased simultaneously are questions of structural transformation and social change, grounded in the voices and articulations of communities that are disenfranchised.

Technologies and Health

As noted in the introductory paragraph, technology has served as the foundation of globalization processes, consolidating power in the hands of transnational capital through the creation of network infrastructures that serve as the foundations for the exchange of information, knowledge, capital, goods, labor, and services. The mobility of capital across global boundaries is made possible by technology, connecting investors to innovations, raw materials, labor, and markets. Technologies are central in commodity flows, pricing structures, and investments into commodities, and the circulation of profits extracted from the global transactions in commodities. In this sense, then, the effects on health that have been discussed in the context of the health-enhancing role of technologies needs to be situated in conversation with the health-depleting and health-threatening roles of technologies.

Technology and Economy

Technology lies at the heart of globalization processes, creating pathways and networks of flows for goods, services, capital, and labor. Technology enables the accelerated rates of production in the global economy, and simultaneously catalyzes pathways for the circulation of global products and services in new and spatially distributed markets across the globe. Moreover, technology occupies the center stage of global production processes, enabling communication, coordination, and exchange across global spaces, simultaneously consolidating resources in the hands of the owners of capital. In other words, technology has formed the cornerstone of globalization processes, playing a key role in shaping the inequalities globally and in the deployment of processes that extract resources from the peripheries and accumulate wealth among the elite actors globally.

Technology also is central to the global creation of new markets. TNCs reach out to markets of new consumers in emerging markets through technologically mediated platforms that create networks for circulating commoditized affinities. Social networking platforms and other forms of digital media become resources for the creation of global value chains shaped in the form of specific consumer desires, disseminated and exchanged through new communication technologies. Sites such as Amazon and eBay emerge as online marketplaces of global exchange. The new media web also emerges as the web of consumption, circulating product affinities and values that are central to the capitalist logic. Technology mediates the advertising, promoting, marketing, and movements of commodities produced under oppressive labor conditions in the global South and in specially designated economic zones across the globe where labor and environmental legislations are weakened in order to generate the optimal conditions for maximum return on investments.

Financialization, Communication Technologies, and Health

The advent of information communication technologies enabled real-time financial transactions in world financial markets, thus integrating these markets in a global financial network, connecting them, and enabling online transactions in globally distributed, interconnected, and intertwined networks. The global ascendance of neoliberal governance is tied to the power of U.S. financial capital to dictate the terms of global financial flows, working through the power of the U.S. state exerted both directly and indirectly (Panitch & Konings, 2009), and in collaboration with global transnational elites (Robinson, 2004). The financialization of the globe is accomplished through the powerful role of communication technologies in creating value through information inequities, assigning value to products and services, and in circulating these values in technologically mediated global networks of financial power (Guvenen, 2013). Inequities in information flows form the basis of the further consolidation of power in the hands of the global financial elite, enabled by the role of technology in facilitating information exchange, financial transactions, and transfer of resources (Guvenen, 2013; Vitali, Glattfelder & Battiston, 2011). The flow of financial value is tied to the quality of information that flows in technology networks, pointing to the elements of quantity, accuracy, timing, quality, and credibility of information that constitute financial decision support systems (Guvenen, 2013).

Instruments such as credit derivatives and lending work toward the consolidation of resources among the owners of capital even as low- and middle-income families are rendered devoid of basic resources of life because of their lack of access to the information-driven financialized economy (Vitali et al., 2011). The financialization of the globe, constituted in the networked communication infrastructures built on information technologies, is a key feature of global neoliberal transformation, accompanied by the manifestation of large-scale inequalities brought about by the extreme concentration of power and wealth in the hands of the global elite, lack of access to basic resources among the poor, low wages, and the growing unemployment among youth, the impoverishment of the middle classes, and the weakening of social securities. Networks of communication across global spaces play essential roles in speculations, assignment of value, and financial transactions. Investors, speculators, and financiers work with real-time data across global markets in their financial transactions that are carried out over information technology networks.

Take, for instance, the emergence and global dominance of Bloomberg as a financial information provider. The emergence of Bloomberg as a global leader in the business information industry is tied to the development of a technological innovation in the form of a consolidated system with easy-to-use terminals and labels with familiar financial terms, two flat-panel monitors to allow ease of information use, a built-in analysis button, and system capacity to compute alternative scenarios and perform longitudinal analyses of historical data (Lee, 2014). Also Bloomberg added information and purchasing services meant to complement the personal lives of traders so traders could buy items such as flowers, clothing, and jewelry; get information about products such as wines; and search through real estate listings. The technology innovated at Bloomberg formed the basis of the financialization processes, creating value and locating this value within the networks of capital. The value generated by technologies of control is circulated through technology networks. Large corporate owners and managers exert their influence through technologies, working through unequal information flows to add extractive value in the form of profits for transnational corporations.

Technologies and Labor

Many of the technologies of capital today are produced in high-tech factories across global spaces where environmental and labor regulations are fairly weak, creating the environments for maximum profit extraction for technology-driven transnationals and for manufacturing units that produce these technologies. The labor that goes into the production of global technologies becomes increasingly invisible as the technologies get miniaturized, simultaneously erasing the discursive possibilities for engaging with questions of worker rights, worker abuse, and worker health (Chan & Ngai, 2010; Pun & Smith, 2005). That these technologies require large investments of labor must therefore remain erased from communicative spaces in order to ensure authoritarian structures for maximum profit extraction through strict regimens that discipline labor. For instance, Apple partners with the manufacturing units of Foxconn housed in special economic zones in the Pearl and Yangtze River Deltas of China, where workers work under strict disciplinary control to produce the iPhone technology in assembly lines (Pun, 2005a, 2005b; Pun & Chan, 2004; Pun & Smith, 2005; Qiu, 2012). The military-style management of labor processes accompanied by unaccountable flexible hiring and firing practices at Foxconn are integral to the extractive information technology economies of global transnationals such as Apple, depicting the collaborative relationship between local manufacturing units and transnational hegemony in the global flow of labor.

Erased simultaneously from the miniaturized and automated stories of Apple products are the narratives of work that go into the assembly lines that produce these slick Apple products such as the iPhone. Workers have minimal rights in these production zones and don't have opportunities to participate in collective bargaining processes. The health effects of the long hours of work on these assembly lines are manifest in workplace injuries, depression, and suicide (Qiu, 2012). Qiu (2012) draws attention to the labor processes of material production, where the labor of the worker is programmed into the computer as the precise movement of specific body parts, thus setting objectives, deliverables, and goals to be achieved by "'programmed' parts of the industrial machine" (p. 175). Workplace injuries such as loss of fingertips depict the unarticulated health effects of the "weightless" and "fingertip" economies of global technology flows.

The onset of the movement of Chinese labor into electronics manufacturing from heavy industry was catalyzed by a number of state-led interventions that took place simultaneously with the participation of China in WTO. The relaxation of registration policies that accompanied the setting up of the new SEZs saw the vast influx of Chinese youth from rural areas into the manufacturing units, working longer and strictly disciplined hours for lesser and lesser pay. Workers, migrating away from rural areas and away from their families, live in mass scale dormitories, in close proximity to their places of work. Their private spaces of everyday living are just as much under surveillance as are the spaces of work. The physical and mental health effects of these poor working conditions and strict disciplinary control mostly remain unaccounted for. The global financial crisis in 2008 produced the backdrop for twenty million job losses in China in 2009, accounting for 80 percent of the total number of job losses in OECD countries and generating the context for severe worker mistreatment, unpaid wages, and worker exploitation at manufacturing units in SEZs in China. The post-2008 fall of Lehman Brothers was accompanied by the sharp decline in the global demand for consumer electronics, manifesting in dramatic job losses. Foxconn responded to the global crisis by firing 100,000 of its 500,000 workers in mainland China in October 2008, followed by firing another 40,000 workers in December 2008. In the case of the labor processing units in Foxconn, the suicide of a worker in 2009 who had been accused of stealing a cell phone was the first among a series of suicides in Foxconn manufacturing units throughout 2010, drawing global attention to the poor working conditions at the technology manufacturing units.

The negative affective and physical health effects of the exploitative work conditions in the information technology industry expand to the global networks of knowledge economy, information economy, and service economy, embodied in business processing outsourcing centers distributed across global spaces (Mirchandani, 2004). The development and diffusion of technologies that reduce distance and offer accelerated performance are integral to the flexible movement of labor in the global information economy. For instance, as call centers emerged in the global South as spaces for carrying out specific components of information-technology-based jobs such as delivering technical support, youth from middle- and lower-middle-income families in economies across the global South have been drawn in large numbers to these opportunities (Shome, 2006). Working long hours, job stressors, and the temporary nature of jobs are all features of globally distributed call center jobs, which are positioned as fun and energizing spaces of growth economies in mainstream discourses of global flows.

The reversed work hours (night shifts) to meet the needs of the inequitable power terrains situated in the global North; the stressors attached to meeting deliverables on tight timelines; the continuous monitoring of job performance on automated systems that measure volume, flow, call handling times, abandonment rates, and so on; and the casual and temporary nature of work at the call centers all contribute to poor mental and physical health outcomes among call center employees. Work is mediatized through technology, also producing health effects in terms of musculoskeletal pain and visual discomfort, further resulting in long-term health outcomes. Call center employees often report digestive disorders, associated with irregular eating times (Sudhashree, Rohith & Shrinivas, 2005). The economy of the call center operates within the trajectories of a new colonialism where biological cycles and health habits of workers in the global South are invaded by the logics of capital enabled by technologies of communication. Call centers also become the consolidated sites of stress where employees negotiate job burnout as they work extreme shifts, having to meet call volumes that are established as targets. Accelerated performance is shaped by performance-driven evaluation metrics and the corresponding implementation of these metrics in hiring and firing decisions.

Moreover, call center employees perform on jobs that require them to train in accent, cultural sensitivity, and communication skills that cater to consumers/clients often situated in the global North, reproducing the uneven terrains of power within which communication is constituted. Employees at call center locations in India, for instance, take on American identities (in the form of American names and accents), performing these identities in their interactions with their U.S.-based clients, often with the intended goal of having to ensure that the client does not perceive their location in India.

The Health Effects of Technology

As noted in the previous section, using technology over extended periods of time is often associated with negative health effects such as musculoskeletal effects, effects on vision, and neural disorders (Kesavachandran et al., 2006). Moreover, prolonged use of technologies such as computers at work and home reifies a sedentary lifestyle, further being likely to contribute toward chronic diseases such as coronary heart disease and diabetes. Using "fingertip" technologies is likely to result in various forms of fingertip injuries over the long term. "Blackberry thumb," for instance, is a condition that arises from the repeated use of small keyboards on mobile devices (Karim, 2009). The health effects of technology cumulatively accumulate over extended periods of time, through repeated movements in operating the technology.

Technologies such as the internet also emerge as avenues for disseminating both health-promoting (more on health promotion in the next section) as well as health-depleting behaviors (such as addiction to unhealthy behaviors). In instances of both forms of behavior, whether health promoting or health depleting, a commodity is pushed among the target audience through the technology, reifying markets for continually invented innovations. Technology in this sense is complicit in processes of market promotion, creating new wants and finding appropriate markets for delivering these wants through targeted and interactive communication strategies, delivered through precise technologies of communication. Social networking sites such as Facebook emerge as both health-enhancing and health-depleting spaces, working simultaneously to deliver an active networked audience that reproduces the market rationality of Facebook. Social networking sites pose a variety of health concerns, including concerns about privacy, confidentiality, online bullying, and harassment.

The food and beverage industry has adopted social media as key communication channels for creating a consumer base. The U.S. food industry spends US$1.6 billion every year targeting young people (Richardson & Harris, 2011; Yale Rudd Center for Food Policy and Obesity, n.d.). In these multimillion-dollar communication campaigns, Facebook and Twitter have emerged as key channels for reaching out to consumer segments, especially in the youth segment (Powell, Harris & Fox, 2013; Richardson & Harris, 2011). These social and new media channels create new interactive avenues for marketing foods and beverages, with strong potential negative health outcomes. Richardson and Harris (2011), in their content analysis of Facebook campaigns launched by the food and beverage industry, noted that Coca-Cola is the most popular Facebook brand and Starbucks is the third-most popular Facebook brand. Also, the brands Red Bull, Monster, Dr. Pepper, Oreo (number four), Skittles (number eight), Pringles (number eleven), Ferrero Rocher (number fourteen), and Nutella (number sixteen) ranked among the top twenty most popular brands on Facebook. Similarly, Powell et al. (2013) report that food and beverage marketing directed at youth on new media platforms is increasing as reported in 2012 as compared with figures gathered in 2006, with a 50.7 percent increase in new media marketing expenditures.

The cycle of commodity promotion and the networks of circulation of unhealthy products also become avenues for marketing health products, further leveraging the commoditizing functions of new media and contributing to the commodity value of the new media. The commodity values of new media platforms such as Facebook and Twitter increase as both healthy and unhealthy products clamor for "likes," "comments," and "retweets." Self-help programs, exercise regimens, and technology-enabled health-promoting strategies all become avenues for pushing commodities in new markets of consumers, defined around specific health needs. Take, for instance, the sugary-sweet industry of brands such as Coke, Pepsi, and Mountain Dew. The industry aggressively utilizes technology-enabled marketing strategies to reach out to target segments, including segments composed of children. Games, social media strategies, and advertising form key components of a comprehensive strategic messaging repository. Simultaneously, funds are allocated toward developing technology-enabled communication strategies for promoting health behaviors among target segments, including children, with a particular emphasis on countering the messages disseminated by manufacturers of sugary-sweet drinks.

Paradoxically, the health messaging framework also gets co-opted into the messaging strategies of manufacturers of sugary-sweet drinks. For instance, Coke carries out a corporate social responsibility campaign targeting obesity, with critical brand presence of the campaign on the World Wide Web. Health ironically then becomes the market logic for drawing in new consumer segments and for promoting the brand value of Coca-Cola. The "Coming Together" campaign website lists video games, tips on healthy eating, and tips on exercising, as well as interactive features such as games, trackers, and polls. The news section lists a variety of Coca-Cola-partnered active living events such as "A healthier Harlem," "Happy movement: Poland campaign," and "Troops for fitness." The website also presents Coca-Cola-sponsored videos of campaign components, such as "get the ball rolling," which is targeted at promoting active living. An interactive map on the website points to the various geographically distributed campaign events titled under "Coming Together around the World." The Twitter handle of the campaign joins the business goals of Coca-Cola with healthy communities: "A business can only be as healthy as the community it's in. It's about where #community needs meet biz."

In the neoliberal organizing of global lifestyles, new and social media emerge as powerful tools for the dissemination of product narratives, leveraging the interactive and social networking capacities of these media to generate more users and capture greater consumer bases. The Coca-Cola Facebook page has over seventy-five million "likes" and leverages localized storytelling to co-construct the stories of users, posting and sharing their stories about consuming Coke (viewing data from November 5, 2013). Consumers post their stories of drinking Coke along with their images of participating in everyday fun activities with Coke. Coke thus is incorporated into the everyday lives of consumers in the form of user engagement enabled through the interactive storytelling features of new media applications. These stories and images are embedded within images of Coke logos on its Facebook site. The images then serve as spaces for co-constructive storytelling, with users sharing the images, posting their comments, posting additional stories in response in the "Comments" section, and so on, fostering networks of consumption. Interaction and participation are framed within broader narratives of consumer engagement, leveraging the peer and networking influence of new and social media to create new markets, to exert normative influence, and to shape product purchase decisions.

Technologies in Military Interventions

The previous chapter outlined the role of technology as an instrument of military aggression that fundamentally threatens health. New media technologies play pivotal roles on the circulation of images that drum up public opinion in support of imperial invasions, often framed in the language of liberty and freedom. As evidenced in the recent Western invasions of Afghanistan and Iraq, as well as in the Western imperial interventions in Libya and in other nation-states in the Middle East, communication technologies play critical functions as instruments of propaganda in the hands of the power elite, circulating images, narratives, and rhetoric that offer humane justifications for Western imperialism. Images justifying the invasions work on the dominant narratives of the civilizing mission, justifying the invasions as acts of civilizing the primitive spaces that are being invaded. Images of veiled women, honor killings, and Taliban oppression of women circulate every day in mainstream media narratives. The new media have become sites for circulating stories of oppression, generating "likes," "comments," and "shares." Building up to the invasions of Iraq and Afghanistan, imperialism was configured in new forms, with technology offering the wherewithal for reporting propaganda images from the ground.

The embedding of journalists during Operation Iraqi Freedom was one such example of communicative processes that circulated real-time images of war, reproducing the positive affect constituted by guns, artillery, military equipment, and armed soldiers. New media technologies similarly are incorporated into democracy-promotion initiatives with imperial undertones, seeking to work through new media channels to disseminate top-down agendas of global imperial powers. The articulations of technologies as harbingers of democracy, liberty, and freedom continue to reiterate the post–World War II development framework where development agencies such as USAID use the democracy trope to push U.S. economic and geostrategic interests globally.

The aggressive and deleterious health effects of war are further fine-tuned by newer and newer innovations of military technologies that create even greater impact with greater precision. The drones that have formed vital components of the U.S. military program abroad emerge as exemplars of war technologies that threaten human health in the most fundamental ways. The number of civilian casualties produced by these technologies speak to their health-threatening nature. Moreover, the deployment of communication as an inversion works precisely to obfuscate the large-scale deaths in civilian populations caused by such technologies. The language of precise targeting in a war against terror emerges as the narrative account for technologies of war and military.

Health Communication Technologies

As noted throughout the book, starting from the Cold War era development communication work to the neoliberal frameworks of health communication, communication technologies occupy the center stage in health communication in catalyzing change in target populations. Much of health communication conceives of communication as a conduit for diffusing technologies of biomedicine that are seen as innovations. Moreover, technology emerges as the communicative platform, the diffusion of which into target communities would bring about economic growth, development, modernization, and as a consequence better health outcomes. Health communication technologies, thus defined as channels for dissemination of biomedical technologies in recipient communities that are disenfranchised, are foregrounded in the neoliberal structures of health organizing.

The diffusion of technology framework leaves intact the organizing power structures that constitute health inequalities while at the same time suggesting stopgap technological fixes for the poor and the underserved. Erased from the discursive spaces are questions of unequal distribution of resources, the dramatic inequalities in distribution of power, and the role of technologies in exacerbating these power differentials. Also absent are the lived experiences of recipient communities as targets of these technology-based interventions. Empirical evidence is subverted to the taken-for-granted assumptions of techno-determinism, built on the uncharted faith that there must be a technological solution to any problem, fostering market-based rationalities for privatized solutions, private innovations, and private–public partnerships.

Information Communication Technologies for Development (ICT4D)

As noted in the introduction to this chapter, one of the central tenets of the development communication literature conceptualizes technology as an instrument of development. This fetishization of technology is the organizing concept of the ICT4D literature, treating technology diffusion as an instrument of development (Mazzarella, 2010). The "free market" logic of neoliberalism has been mobilized in this literature through the framework of civil society initiatives in partnership with the private sector, especially corporatized networks of telecommunication. Building private technology networks in underserved areas such as in rural communities and in communities living in poverty is seen as a mechanism for addressing larger problems of poverty and inaccess.

The neoliberal logic of technology diffusion sees technology as a universal good that access to which promises to bring about changes in economic access to resources. In spite of the claims of the ICT4D literature regarding the instrumental roles of technology in addressing questions of development, health, and poverty, there remains little conclusive evidence that points convincingly toward such roles played by technology. In contrast, a substantive body of the literature points toward the increasing gaps between the haves and have-nots that are brought about by technology-driven problems. The market mechanisms proposed as solutions continue to reify the existing power differentials, thus maintaining and reproducing large-scale inequalities. Summarizing this position eloquently, Sreekumar (2011, p. 12) notes:

> This new ICT discourse maintains that digital divide is the site of a major unequalizing force in the contemporary world economy. As a corollary, it assumes that this divide could be bridged by supplying more ICTs to developing countries. This would in turn imply the fallacious position that the standard cost-benefit comparisons are irrelevant in the case of ICT projects, since ICTs form the fulcrum of a new paradigm of social and economic development. Accordingly, and with loyalty to these convictions, groupthink admits no failures as a rule; exceptions are when they could be brushed aside as a lag in rectifying training inadequacies, tackling cultural constraints or eliciting political will.

The emphasis on technology solving the overarching structural problems of inequality, poverty, and resource inaccess depicts a form of technology fetishism within neoliberal structures that uncritically accept the power of technology as the leveling field. Technology is seen thus as an equalizer, obtuscating the structural, political, and cultural contexts. When a technology-driven project fails, and this happens often in the global South (Sreekumar, 2011), bureaucrats and technocrats search for some other underlying reason, thus recycling the technological solutions as frameworks for development.

For a variety of projects carried out in the global South, funds deployed into the technologies are not cross-checked against the metrics of poverty and unemployment that the technologies promise to address in project descriptions. Glossy brochures, websites, and communication materials directed at external stakeholders, often for the purpose of generating additional funding and performing the public relations functions for donors, are not really aligned with the metrics of poverty, inequality, and inaccess within communities. Dominant articulations of performance don't really offer measurements that speak to the lofty narratives of poverty alleviation. The voices of local communities, their dreams and aspirations, and their understandings of problems and solutions are erased from the spaces of reporting. Reports, as instruments of neoliberal control, reify the logics of exclusion and marginalization of subaltern communities, reifying stories that are performed toward powerful social actors and elite stakeholders within the academic–civil society–private foundations networks.

Targeting and Message Tailoring

Technologies have been deployed to increase the precision of segmentation and message targeting strategies, directed toward generating greater health outcomes in targeted communities of strategic interest (Glasgow et al., 2004). Technologies ensure campaigns a precise reach into target populations on the basis of the premise of precise data analysis strategies combined with the ability to target audiences through the gathering of intelligent data. Web-based technologies, for instance, are positioned as solutions for delivering targeted health interventions in at-risk communities through the capacity of technologies to offer tailored or customized solutions that meet the needs of targeted audiences. These technologies are seen as more efficient in enabling the segmentation of audiences as compared with the traditional communication channels, such as television, that are seen as having a broader but much less selective reach (Kreuter et al., 2013).

The concepts of targeting and tailoring therefore are seen as tools for aligning the health message with the communicative needs and profile of the audience. The role of health communication research focuses on figuring out the appropriate trait level and the attitudinal, cognitive, and behavioral characteristics that can guide the principles of messaging. The right message delivered through the right technology is expected to bring about the intended change in the target population. E-health interventions targeting specific disease traits segment the population on the basis of certain preconfigured characteristics and develop messages for dissemination on the basis of these characteristics.

Digital Divide and the Solutions of Technology

Digital divide refers to the gaps in access to communication technologies between and within different sectors of the population. Scholars examining digital divide in health contexts describe the correlations between health disparities and digital divide. These observations suggest that those sectors of the population with poorer health outcomes are also more likely to be digitally disenfranchised, with lower levels of access to communication technologies. The solutions proposed in the backdrop of this digital divide literature are solutions that privilege the technologies of access. For instance, NCI launched a number of digital divide projects seeking to address the disparities in cancer and access to communication technologies experienced by communities. The digital divide framework then seeks to build infrastructures of new communication technologies, community-driven technological platforms, and community-based training programs directed at fostering the access, ability, and motivation to use new communication technologies for health purposes.

The overarching logic of the neoliberal framework of health organizing privileges technological remedies while at the same time leaving intact the structural contexts of health disparities. The solutions of technology continue to understand health as being constituted through the use of technology, while at the same time failing to account for the political and economic structures constituting poor health outcomes in underserved communities. Amid the large-scale neoliberal reforms and financialization of the U.S. economy, the rising discourse of health inequalities has been accompanied by a corresponding discourse of cyberinfrastructures, digital divide projects, and information technology capacity building. Paradoxically, the answer to these disparities framed through the lens of technology is not a fundamental transformation in structures, but rather an insistence on behavior change embodied in messages promoting lifestyle change, preventive behaviors, and changes in attitudes and beliefs of target audiences. Consider, for instance, the solution offered by Viswanath (2011, p. S247) in his discussion of addressing communication inequalities, making recommendations such as the following:

> (1) investing in building capacity among disadvantaged communities, groups, and nations to take advantage of cyberinfrastructure; (2) making data more easily accessible and usable; (3) involving end users, especially those serving the underserved, in both designing and deploying the systems; and (4) making the boundaries between producers and consumers of knowledge more porous with an explicit focus on addressing inequalities.

Communication inequalities thus are narrowly conceived as inequalities in distribution of communication technologies of information dissemination. The organizing framework assumes a deficit model, based on the organizing framework of knowledge gap, reifying and circulating the assumption that health inequalities are based on information inequalities. The deficit model offers the overarching framework, suggesting that deficits in top-down information designed by experts result in health inequalities. The techno-deterministic narrative foregrounding technological solutions to health inequalities is well captured in the title of Viswanath's article, "Cyberinfrastructure: An Extraordinary Opportunity to Bridge Health and Communication Inequalities?"

It is also worth noting that the technologies for addressing disparities are predominantly channels of dissemination, sending out strategically created, effective health-promoting messages. In much of the digital divide literature, the roles of technologies as tools of health advocacy and health activism, the constitutive roles of technology in enabling structural transformation, and the roles of technology as resources for collective mobilization against the overarching inequalities in distribution of power and material resources remain unaddressed. The large-scale inequities in distribution of power and inequalities in communicative opportunities for participation are reified through the definition of participation in the ambits of technology, limiting participation to those actors within structures of access and simultaneously devaluing the participation of these that remain beyond the reach of the dominant organizing structures.

Technologies and Participation

In the neoliberal narrative of health governance, technologies are conceptualized as enablers of participatory processes (Harris et al., 2013). The narrative of technology-enabled democracy frames technology as the harbinger of democratic politics, reiterating the often-repeated narrative of early development communication interventions that conceived technology as an instrument for modernization. Consider the following depiction offered by Harris et al. (2013, p. 488):

> A metamorphosis toward participatory health creates mass potential for autonomy and confident self-maintenance using secure technology tools and health promotion methods. Health IT can also facilitate efficient information seeking and the creation of digital social networks. This potential, especially in the context of the significant public financial investment underway to increase the adoption of health IT and making it an explicit part of the health communication topic area for Healthy People 2020.

The positivist portrayal of health information technology as the harbinger of participation reifies a neoliberal narrative of health, pushing forth ideas of efficiency and effectiveness as the anchors of health communication. Participation in health is fostered through and constituted by technology. Participation is constituted in its relationship to efficient health care, with information technology enabling the efficient delivery, efficient information seeking, and development of health-efficient digital social networks.

Health decisions and health policies are thus articulated in a positive narrative, with the organizing role of communication technologies in fostering spaces for participation, engagement, and dialogue. Technologies thus are seen as enablers of democratic processes, as channels for promoting community participation and engagement. The participatory spaces fostered by technology are seen as democratizing decision-making processes, fostering opportunities for public participation, consultation, and dialogue. It is worth noting that NGOs emerge as representatives of communities in these technology-enabled participatory processes.

The communicative heuristic that community representation equates to representation by NGOs lies at the heart of the constructions of technology-enabled participatory processes. Worth noting are the requirements of literacy and technological capacity as the markers of participation. In an NGO-driven technology-enabled participatory space, the ability to access the necessary communicative resources that are required for participation in civil society processes play crucial roles in shaping the processes and textures of participation. For instance, Harris et al. (2013) offer the example of the decision-making processes in Healthy People 2020 as an exemplar of IT-enabled participatory and transparent decision-making processes in health policy making. The exemplars of participatory channels included workgroup meetings and consultations, a public comment website, a public meeting of the advisory committee, and a request for public comment published in the *Federal Register*. Worth noting here is the very nature of public participation and technology-enabled participation that is tied to privilege, technological access, and technological literacy. Questions such as "Who participates in the online public commentaries?," "Who participates in the public comments requests published in the *Federal Register*?," "Who participates in the workgroup meetings, and who is invited to these meetings?" remain outside the discursive space. In this framework, making a public comment website open to the public is participatory to the extent that community members have access to the technology, are interested and able to participate in the public comment channels on the web, are aware of the public comment option available on the web, and are able to navigate the public comment channels on the web. The notion of technology-enabled participation in sharing public comments on a website as being the equivalent of participation obfuscates the ongoing research that points to digital divides in access and substantive population-wide differences in the motivation and ability to use online technologies of participation. Participation and transparency thus are imbricated upon the principles of exclusion, with technology emerging as a marker of exclusion. To build technology literacy programs, technological capacity such as broadband capacity, and technology-enabled participatory infrastructures as solutions of public participation strategically deploys an idea of participation that limits it to the dominant structures and to the social classes that fit within the ambits of citizenship as defined within these structures.

Moreover, as in the example of the participatory processes working toward the agenda-setting function for Healthy People 2020, the ambits of participation enabled by new technologies are defined within the agenda-setting functions of the dominant power structures. The constraints imposed on participation ensure that the fundamentally unhealthy structures remain intact, as health information technologies are framed as solutions working toward promoting stronger health-oriented beliefs, attitudes, and behaviors. Participation, framed within the ambits of individual behavior and lifestyle modification, is defined and limited in scope by the objectives of the dominant actors. Given the biases within these e-participatory structures toward dominant communicative skill sets that are required to participate, participation is structured within elite circles within communities that have the communicative access to occupy the technology-enabled spaces. Community thus becomes synonymous with NGOs even as most NGO workers serving the community either reside outside the community or are elite members from within the community. The community, understood as a monolith represented in the participation of the key actors who participate in the e-participation forum, is thus shaped within the definitional parameters of the technology.

Websites, E-Health, and Mobile Health

Resources such as websites, e-health infrastructures, and mobile health platforms reproduce the narrative of technology-enabled health, constituting new technologies for the delivery of health information, prevention messages, social support, and other forms of health communication solutions. Technologies such as websites, text messages, and mobile applications are seen as platforms for the delivery of health information and for the circulation of health appeals promoting preventive behaviors. These resources are also integral to the logics of commercialization, with health information resources such as WebMD serving as channels for the advertising of health products. Information in commercial interests is often framed as public interest information, obfuscating the line between health information and health advertising. DTC advertisements are formatted within structures of health information, thus misleading potential consumers by blurring the lines between information and advertising.

E-health, broadly conceived as the delivery of health information online and the dissemination of persuasive health messages, is constituted within a narrative of patient empowerment through technology. Consider the following depiction of e-health communication put forth by Suggs and Ratzan (2012, p. 257):

> Recent trends in e-health communication give health consumers more control and power regarding how, what, and when they receive and provide information about health. Web technology pushed and continues to push the boundaries that health communication professionals used to control. Society's technological progress presents an opportunity for developing health literacy—advancing knowledge and skills while reducing complexity such that individuals and health providers can make appropriate decisions.

The image of the empowered patient controlling information flows through technology and shaping the relevant information that would enable effective participation in the marketplace lies at the heart of neoliberal health communication. Literacy is framed within the ambits of the dominant structure, configured as knowledge of skills situated in relationship to mainstream articulations of health. The active patient that is empowered and literate participates in making effective health decisions and in making healthy choices amid a gamut of health options.

In my own early work and in the works of scholars working with the construct of technologically mediated health information seeking, the activated health consumer is highly motivated and able to enact sophisticated health choices, participating actively in seeking health information, optimizing health beliefs, developing healthy attitudes, participating in community organizations to optimize health, and engaging in health-promoting behaviors. Consider the following depiction offered by Suggs and Ratzan (2012, p. 255):

> With improved access to health information (e.g., via the Internet and the mass media), along with a growing level of medical sophistication among lay persons, patients today are rapidly evolving into "health-competent consumers," taking an active role in their own health and health care, and demanding safe and more effective health care solutions.

The issues, topics, and objects of health knowledge within this framework are limited to knowledge about individual behaviors and lifestyles such as eating healthy, exercising, and so on, reifying the dominant structures that shape health as individual decision making. Absent from the discursive spaces shaped by new communication technologies of health promotion are questions about dominant health structures, the unequal organizing of these structures, and the inequities that result from these structures.

Social media, as networked technologies of communication, are understood within this broader structure of e-health communication as channels for disseminating health messages. Research on social media use patterns in the health context foreground strategies for measuring social media effects, mapping out dissemination patterns on social media, and developing research-driven strategies for the dissemination of messages on social media. The study of social networks is framed within the functions of message delivery and message dissemination, leveraging network structures and communication flows within networks to diffuse innovations (Valente, 2011). New technologies of diffusion in neoliberal governance of health recycle the traditional development narratives of diffusion of innovations, embodying the fundamentals of modernization and behavior change through participation, albeit repackaged in a narrative of technology-enabled participatory communication.

Mobile health applications are conceptualized as low-cost mechanisms for disseminating health information. The delivery of health information is tied to the development of mobile infrastructures and mobile technologies with access to technology being linked to public–private partnerships. Public investments in building mobile infrastructures and subsidies in private mobile phone infrastructures are framed within the ambits of health promotion, while simultaneously obfuscating the commercial contexts of mobile phone penetration. For instance, the Grameen phone as a tool for disseminating health information is also an instrument for serving the commercial interests of Grameen. The Grameen platform not only disseminates health information but also various other kinds of strategic communication promoting products.

Worth interrogating in these e-health interventions are the paradoxical roles of technologies in constituting the very threats to health that are targeted through interventions. Consider, for instance, e-health interventions targeting the epidemic of diabetes. Obfuscated in this framework of e-health as a solution to diabetes are the fundamental threats to health that are posed by technology-dependent lifestyles and the amount of time individuals spend with their screens. The global shifts in lifestyles, in patterns of work, and in the nature and amount of exercising a person gets in a day are constituted by the global penetration of technologies and the role of technologically mediated lives, especially among the global middle classes. Health-promoting websites urging children to exercise erase the essential irony of persuading a child to exercise delivered through a screen. With children increasingly spending their time on new media technologies and the health threats that are constituted by these patterns of behaviors constituted around technologies, e-health interventions depict an essential communicative inversion written into the structures of neoliberal health organizing.

Technologies of Surveillance and Control

Technologies of health are constituted not only in technologies for delivering strategic health communication messages but also in technologies of measurement that place the body under surveillance. The human body becomes a source of data captured through smart devices, continually placing the body as the site of data generation. Innovations on smart devices emphasize mobility, accuracy of measurement, convenience, tasks performed, and so on. Smart technologies incorporated into mobile devices and watches offer the next generation of personalized data capture and data feedback on behaviors such as walking and exercising. These smart devices, often connected to websites and training programs, work through feedback mechanisms to promote and support health behaviors, leveraging the capacity of new technologies to tailor health-promoting messages.

Smart technologies are seen as offering efficient and effective feedback mechanisms on behavior. The logics of efficiency are circulated as the prevailing logic, with an emphasis on individual ownership and responsibility. The emphasis on the individual operates on the logic of optimizing the feedback mechanisms provided to the individual to enable behavior change and behavior maintenance. Models such as the stages of change model coupled with smart technologies create effective mechanisms for delivering effective messages to the individual health consumer. The emphasis placed on the individual operates within the neoliberal framework of health organizing.

Worth noting are the collaborative relationships between smart technologies of surveillance and consumer marketing, with smart data operating as market data for targeting and strategic communication. The data gathered on bodily performance, movement, and everyday health practices are also connected with and fed to commercial marketing and market research companies, turning the body into a site of targeting with invitations to consume. Behaviors, understood in the realm of health, are connected to a range of other behaviors, constituting the individual subject as a consumer. Advertisements for diet products and exercise regimens exploit the data on consumer behavior and everyday practices to fine-tune targeting and messaging strategies.

The Technology Paradox

The technological determinism of neoliberal governance is rooted in the pervasiveness of technocratic solutions and in the positioning of technology as the solution to global health problems. This primordial focus on technology finds continuity from the technologically deterministic model of development communication that foregrounded the role of communication technologies in bringing about social change, forming the basis of social change interventions that were targeted at disseminating these technologies across the globe. The formulation of problems is positioned as the absence or the lack of technology, to which then the solution of technology is pushed through a variety of targeted communication interventions, well captured in the key formulations of the widely accepted diffusion of innovations framework in communication studies. Most communication studies operating within this framework begin with the assumption that the technology as an innovation is a solution to a given problem configuration, and then examine the communicative processes, strategies, and stages through which the innovation is disseminated or adopted in the wider population.

This reductionist framing of technology as a solution to human problems does not attend to broader questions of the societal-level effects of the technology or the unintended and side effects of the technology, as well as its broader social, cultural, political, and economic consequences. The diffusion of innovations framework that formed the cornerstone of communication for social change therefore operated on the assumption that technologies were instrumental in the catalysis of development processes, without attending to the broader contexts of technology adoption, the broader effects produced by the rapid adoption of a technology-driven worldview, and the larger consequences of technologies. Under neoliberal governance, the emphasis on technology has been consolidated as a source of power in the hands of the owners of capital, turning technology-based solutions into new products that can be directed at consumers, creating and reproducing new markets for the capital-intensive technologies.

The creation of new markets and the simultaneous creation of new problems are integral to the accelerated production of technological solutions and the rapid dissemination of these solutions in global markets across geographic spaces. Take, for instance, the current problem of climate change and the technologically deterministic framing of this problem around the language of sustainability, climate adaptation, and environmental consciousness. What lies at the root of human-produced climate change processes is the narrowly reductionist technologically deterministic worldview that has produced a wide variety of unintended effects that were initially not conceived of as potential effects of the technology. However, because of the reductionist nature of a technologically determined worldview, the accelerated adoption of these technologies across global markets remained oblivious to a wide variety of side effects on the environment that were being generated by these technologies. Yet as the global community works toward finding solutions to a predominantly technology-induced problem of climate change, the market-driven elite structures of neoliberal governance return to the technologically determined framework to find solutions.

The inherent paradox of technology in neoliberal governance lies in the precise framing of technological solutions as the predominant solutions to problems that in essence have been caused by the rapid diffusion of a reductionist worldview that has been inattentive to the potential side effects of the technologies being diffused through neoliberal structures. The market-driven logic of neoliberal governance works toward finding new products, designs, and deliverables, which, in turn, then are intrinsically connected with the creation of new markets for capital. For example, the positioning of biotechnology as a solution to climate change processes pushes a technologically reductionist worldview, oblivious to the diversity of the pathways of adaptive agricultural practices in place in rural communities across the globe, the locally specific solutions to climate change processes, and local adaptation processes. Moreover, in pushing a corporate-driven profit-based model of agricultural technology as a universal form of adaptation to climate change processes, the biotechnology framework reiterates the same fundamental mistakes of technological shortsightedness that are intrinsic to the technology adoption processes that produce climate change and threaten the environment.

Similarly, within the context of health care, the framing of technologically driven health systems as revolutions in health care remains oblivious to the side effects and unintended consequences of these technologies for health care, especially within the context of the problem of the increasing price of health care. Solutions such as e-health, patient-centered care, and electronic medical records (EMRs) are put out as solutions that save health care costs through the promise of better management even as these solutions are themselves cost-intensive. Much like other adoptions of technologies as innovations that take for granted the likely effects of the technology, the claims regarding the role of technology in reducing costs often remains untested. The assumption that the technology will automatically reduce cost and increase efficiency once adopted across the globe drives large investments into research and development, and subsequent diffusion, without appropriate and culturally grounded testing of the technology through pilot projects in the specific local context. The development and implementation of health technologies is shaped by the promise of new markets for these technologies that require expenditure even as these technologies are themselves put forth as instruments for saving costs for health care. Often absent from the assumptions of technological efficiency are questions regarding the costs of technology development, the costs of dissemination and system modification, the costs of training, and the likely unintended management roles that are introduced by the technology. Once again, a fundamental paradox in practice forms the basis of the technological revolution that is introduced as a cost-cutting innovation. The effectiveness of neoliberal governance rests precisely on this paradox, in the unaccounted for, unverified, and untested assumptions about the effective and efficient working of technology as an innovative solution across global markets.

This lack of attentiveness to evidence forms the basis of neoliberal governance as innovations are introduced into global markets on the basis of the premises of efficiency and effectiveness without needing to be held accountable to the material manifestations of the claims that are circulated as justifications for technological innovations. The communicative turn in interpretive frames that disregards the material bases of articulations works hand in hand with the neoliberal organizing of global spaces, creating global markets for commodities and technologies and simultaneously disregarding evidence, observations, and material structures. Understanding the "technology paradox" as intrinsic to the hegemony of technology calls for health communication scholarship that makes visible the interpretations of and lived experiences with technologies.

Conclusion

If one of the key characteristics of neoliberal globalization of health is the emphasis on military interventions, the other salient feature of global health structures is the fetish of technology. Technology is the instrument for better health within the neoliberal structures of health, often devoid of systematic evaluations of the potential fit of the technology with community experiences and without the participation of community members in the designing of the technology. Technology fosters avenues for new technology, thus circulating a market for innovations, feeding into the capitalist structures of profiting. Technology, narrowly conceived as the predominant framework of solutions within neoliberal capitalism, works toward serving the agendas of the power elite while simultaneously obfuscating the participatory opportunities for the resource-poor sectors of the globe. The performance of technology-enabled participation reifies the digital divide, offering the illusion of participation as a public relations strategy. Decisions ultimately are made by experts far removed from communities, with accountability being driven toward donors.

CHAPTER EIGHT

EPILOGUE: NEOLIBERAL HEALTH AND ALTERNATIVES

Recently, I participated in a global public affairs forum held at a five-star hotel in the metropole where one of the team of presenters was a consulting team from a globally reputed multinational consulting organization, working in collaboration with a global food support organization and a number of private partnerships to address food insecurity in the global South, capturing the effectiveness of the program in well-executed and eyeball-capturing PowerPoint slides. The team, composed of MBAs from reputed global universities, discussed the success of its model of development in a country located in the global South, pointing to the success of public–private partnerships as catalysts for social change processes. Intrigued by the data that suggested the wonder and gratitude of the local people in receiving the intervention, when I asked the team leader if she had indeed traveled to this community and experienced the wonder of the recipients firsthand, I was told that there was no need for the expert team to travel to the location as there were local NGOs who were the local experts and who were carrying out the work locally.

This displacement/removal of the "expert" from sites of social change that are framed as passive recipients in gratitude for the social change solutions designed by these experts located in air-conditioned rooms in the global North/West depicts the power of neoliberalism as an organizing framework of global health/development communication, manufacturing and circulating a social class of change makers who fundamentally profit from the business of social change bolstered on a racist logic of imperial control, irresponsibility, and lack of commitment to communities at the grassroots level. In the careless search of target communities dispersed across the globe, intervention planners map out data, conduct needs assessments, plan a few short trips, carry out interventions from a distance, and then write up reports from a distance as well, captured in the certainties of means, standard deviations, and p values. These reports register the social change products and become the instruments for further recycling the logic of altruism, satisfying the funder and becoming tools to be used for generating more funds for future campaigns. The carelessness of this dominant framework of health communication is reflected in the absence of a long-term commitment to the community (with most research reporting short campaign cycles), the erasure of community voices from local spaces of articulation, the episodic nature of interventions, and the disappearance of local communities as sites of accountability. The irresponsibility of the neoliberal framework is normalized because of the fundamental absence of local community structures of accountability, instead relying on far-removed numeric representations that speak to the effectiveness of the campaign. One of the communicative inversions in the participatory social change processes in neoliberal health organizing is this basic absence of accountability to local communities within a grand narrative that advertises widely stories of local participation, accountability, democracy, and transparency, precisely to carry out top-down expert-driven interventions that benefit the status quo. For instance, a variety of World Bank-funded community-based participatory programs are integral to the logic of neoliberal hegemony, positioning the state in opposition to a utopian articulation of the community and doing so to support neoliberal policies of reducing taxes on wealth and income, weakening state-based public health infrastructures, and weakening public welfare programs. Moreover, the language of participation has been incorporated into the privatization of the grassroots in the form of various public-private partnerships couched in the language of democracy.

The teams of experts, albeit multicultural and diverse, are nevertheless elite teams that derive their class power from the distance between the experts and the recipient communities they target. What appears as the inauthenticity of such consulting-driven social change work directed at delivering prescriptive solutions for the global South is precisely the source of power for the neoliberal model of expertise based on the language of empirical/objective distance. The colored representatives on the consulting team indeed represent the face of global social change work, communicating a facade of diversity and multiculturalism, whereas the knowledge structures inhabited by such consulting teams are precisely the structures of West-centric knowledge production that seek to deliver solutions for subaltern communities in the global South on the basis of objective expertise located at far-removed global centers. Ironically, questions of validity, reliability, meaningfulness of data, criteria that are otherwise paraded as the criteria of the post-positivist development model, are obfuscated in the charts and tables that have minimal to no local community accountability. Did the local community find the intervention to be successful? What are the metrics that are most relevant to the local community? How was the campaign interpreted within the cultural contexts of the local community? What are the experiences of local community members? These questions are typically absent from journal articles and reports documenting campaign effectiveness. In such fetishized forms of social change tourism designed and configured within the white liberal structures of the global North, the experts parading the neoliberal solutions have little to no idea of the lived experiences of the targeted communities and often have very little to no interaction with local community members. Culture emerges within this neoliberal model as a marker of the "other" that stands in the way of the universalized logic of the intervention; culturally sensitized messages addressing cultural barriers are seen as pathways for increasing the effectiveness and efficiency of health interventions (see for instance, Bresnahan et al., 2007; Kreuter et al., 2013). The deep-rooted underlying values guiding culturally sensitive health promotion interventions are often Western values framed within universal logics, while the interventions are couched within the superficial markers of culture drawn from expert-driven scales often rooted in the West. For instance, Bresnahan et al. (2007) measure individualistic and collectivistic values in addressing cultural barriers to organ donation, thus treating culture as reflected in superficial measurement of individualism and collectivism while simultaneously obfuscating the fundamental cultural values underlying organ donation. Also worth noting here is the Euro-US-centrism of constructs such as individualism-collectivism that are deployed as measures of culture.

The snippet of the interactions presented in this introduction depicts the organizing power of neoliberalism that rules through expertise located at a distance at the centers of global power in the metropole. The "elsewhere" of global capitalism emerges as the precise point of discussion in the networks of global power, emerging in PowerPoint slides and case studies discussed by the transnational elite, representing various configurations of private–public partnerships and culturally sensitive interventions. Increasingly, in a climate where the narrative of local participation in self-governance emerges as an appeal to democratic development, it is worth noting that the agendas, directives, and key decisions of health and development are very much located among networks of experts located in the centers of power in the global North who only network with each other, not with the targeted communities that must remain as codified voices, captured images, and statistical outcomes of knowledge, attitude, and behavior (KAB) surveys. Moreover, the taken for granted assumptions embodied in these elite networks reproduce the status quo by focusing attention on individual behavior change through the development of effective culturally-sensitive messages while simultaneously obfuscating the structural contexts of health. Forums such as Public Affairs meetings, WEF, and NGO meet-ups emerge as spaces for circulating expert knowledge and establishing the credibility of such knowledge as solutions to global problems, often circulating the very same elite-directed solutions that constitute the underlying reasons for global problems. The participatory capacity of communities are often challenged within these top-down frameworks of development, based on the Western notions of development predicated on the linear model of modernization and economic growth.

In neoliberal structures of global organizing, participation emerges as a strategic management resource for managing projects on the ground, driven by top-down agendas and strategies shaped by experts sitting at centers of power and disseminating technologies conceived and designed in the North. The organizing of neoliberalism is a political economy of expertise, where teams of experts are incentivized to carry out unsustainable interventions in distant locales, without local accountability and local decision making, and carried out in short time frames driven by narrowly defined expert-driven metrics of effectiveness and efficiency. These solutions to global health leave intact the structures of power and in turn reify the logics of neoliberalism by deploying health as a category for creating new markets globally, situating the delivery of health as a mix of marketing and management functions, delivered through public–private partnerships (Ramon, 2008; Rodgers, 2001). Technological solutions are privileged, with an "app" for every health problem. Elite MBA degrees on health and development management offered at elite universities become sites of disciplining and training in expertise, albeit purchased at high costs and directed at mass-producing the next generation of social entrepreneurs and experts who will create the new technological solutions to global health problems, which typically are part of the very structures of neoliberalism that threaten human health and well-being across global contexts (Chandrasekhar & Ghosh, 2001; Dutta, 2011; Rampton & Stauber, 2011; Unwin, 2009).

The political economy of entire industries of information technology for development, health and development communication campaigns, knowledge management functions, and multicultural health promotion solutions, including the salaries of development and health staff, the costs of training programs, and the high profits generated by academic degrees targeting to train potential workers in health, development, and social change communication, is formulated on the very logics of portrayals of the poor and the marginalized as the passive recipients of interventions designed to target them. The multicultural landscape of neoliberal interventionism turns local culture as a decipherable site that must be rendered transparent and subsequently targeted through culturally responsive/adaptive strategies. Culture emerges as a guiding category, married to the economy, drawing funding resources and expert teams to guide the development of knowledge that would address the cultural barriers. In the recent example of Ebola, for instance, cultural teams of experts are employed to figure out the local burial practices and develop appropriate messaging strategies for addressing these burial practices in the context of Ebola (Hewlett & Amola, 2003). Such constructions of culture in the dominant framework erase the opportunities of participation of local communities in processes of decision making and interpretation. The contemporary ascendance of culture as an instrument of neoliberal interventions obfuscates the threats of erasure of cultural understandings, local voices, and local cultural understandings of health and well-being in the face of culturally sensitive interventions that have been designed to co-opt culture for the purposes of effective message delivery. Surface level features such as depicting an African American family in a culturally sensitive healthy eating campaign targeting African Americans erase the histories and contexts of race, food, and politics experienced by African American communities at the margins of a racist and classist health care system (Dutta, 2006, 2007, 2008).

Through the analysis offered through the various sections of the book, we witness the large gaps between the rhetoric of development communicated in messages of neoliberal health organizing and the lived experiences of individuals, households, and communities living at the global margins. Part of the reason underlying this gap is the very structuring of health communication within the organizing frameworks of neoliberalism, embodying neoliberal values that translate into individually based health communication interventions directed by experts in the global North/West. The dominant framework of health communication campaigns, for instance, embodies the neoliberal logic with its emphasis on the individual, targeting individual-level beliefs, attitudes, and behaviors and oblivious to the structural features that constitute health. The theorizing of culture within this framework turns culture into an individual-level variable, marked as a barrier to the diffusion of the intervention (Rogers, 1973, 1983). As experts who are trained in the project of neoliberalism and who depend upon the expansion of neoliberal organizing principles to new markets in the global South to sustain their salaries, health communicators are incentivized to recycle the dominant categories of health, recycling the individual-level framework of behavior modification.

Part of the problem therefore is the underlying ideology of health communication that is embedded within neoliberal principles and that leaves unquestioned the techno-deterministic assumptions that guide global health solutions (Barker, K., 2004; Rogers, 1962, 1973, 1983; Rogers & Svenning, 1969). In this model, experts derive the false confidence that they can somehow develop the wherewithal to travel into a culture or a community (often for short frames of times, a phenomenon of "academic tourism"), prescribe individual-level solutions embodied in communication technologies and intervention messages, and, in the process, circulate the rhetoric of lifting the targeted community out of misery. This naiveté is integral to the culture of expertise built into neoliberalism, with coteries of experts being deployed across global boundaries in implementing top-down health solutions leveraging participatory tools. Solutions such as microcredit lending and the *Grameen Bank* emerge as solutions to health, without really attending to the lived experiences of communities experiencing the interventions (Muhammad, 2009), the structural injustices experienced in the communities, and the marginalizing impacts of the proposed interventions. In this sense, the ideology of neoliberalism achieves its hegemony with minimal engagement with evidence, often couched in empty public relations messages celebrating the virtue of the market, economic growth, and trickle-down economics. In instances where the evidence is indeed presented, it is cast aside as a caveat or as an exception in order to continue circulating the logic of neoliberalism as the solution to health and development. Discussions of neoliberalism are bracketed as polemic, thus reifying the hegemony of individual-level behavior change as the solution to poor health and health risks, albeit with a cursory nod to the structural contexts of health and well-being.

A set of key threads flow through the analysis offered in the book. These threads attend to the intersections of the symbolic and the material in the constructions of health (Artz, 2006), depicting the ways in which culture and communication are structured by organizing processes as well as the various elements of organizing that work through the fabrics of culture and communication to shape both micro- as well as macro-level structures. In this section, we briefly revisit the key points in the literature, seeking to understand the ways in which these themes work within the broader framework of neoliberal organizing of health. A summative reading of these key arguments shaping the neoliberal structures of health organizing provides the backdrop for suggesting alternative imaginations for health communication.

Communicative Inequality

One of the themes that is evident through the various structures of global organizing is the centrality of communicative inequality in constituting health inequalities (Narayan, 1999a, 1999b, 2000). A key argument put forth in the book attends to the mutually constitutive relationship between communicative and health inequalities, noting the positioning of health inequalities amid inequalities of communication processes and differentials in the flow of power. Transforming entrenched patterns of health inequalities is therefore tied to the structural transformations that need to be brought about in communicative systems and processes, fostering spaces of democratic participation of the grassroots that are not co-opted by top-down forms of interventions, shaped in the language of participatory democracy. Technology-centric solutions of health communication, based on imaginations of the information superhighway or cyberinfrastructure (see for instance Viswanath, 2011), continue to reproduce these inequities by leaving intact the broader structural patterns that constitute the inequalities.

Based on the ethnographic fieldwork and community-driven collaborative projects conducted in the framework of the culture-centered approach to health communication (Dutta, 2008), analyses of neoliberal communicative spaces depict the discursive inequalities that constitute (im)possibilities of participation, bringing forth the specific communicative strategies that erase subaltern participatory opportunities even as the language of multiculturalism and subaltern participation emerge as the dominant language of neoliberalism. A critical interrogation of these dominant narratives of participation point toward the co-optive processes that frame participation within monolithic agendas dictated by global power structures, often turning subaltern communities into sites/resources for extraction, exploitation, and profiteering (Dutta & Pal, 2010). Communicative inequalities are reproduced through the political economy of expertise, where experts, often paid by TNCs to lend their voice, serve as gatekeepers of knowledge and the voices of knowledge in the public sphere (Rampton & Stauber, 2001). Inversion of these inequalities, therefore, is also the inversion of inequalities in processes of recognition and representation.

Communicative Inversions

Communicative inversions are the reversal of communication, where symbolic representations refer to markers that are the opposite of the material bases of patterns, relationships, and outcomes. For instance, a fundamentally health-threatening TNC operation is communicatively inverted as health promoting through the use of language, the deployment of specific frames, and the emphasis on particular narrowly selected metrics. Communicative inversions are essential to neoliberal logics of growth, with the portrayals of growth as essential to better health and well-being in spite of the evidence that interrogates this taken-for-granted logic and suggests otherwise. Communication accelerates and recirculates the growth narrative globally, putting forth an unhealthy and blind faith in growth, greater production, and greater consumption. Public relations campaigns, expert-driven knowledge production processes, think tanks, and NGOs consistently work on disseminating the growth narrative, simultaneously erasing questions regarding the limits of/to growth, the threats to health posed by processes of continuous production and consumption, and the fundamentally toxic nature of an overzealous and uncritical commitment to growth. Front groups, paid for by TNCs, offer good examples of communicative inversions, where the facade of representation differs dramatically from the underlying agendas served by these groups. The oil industry recruits front groups that position themselves as environmental activist groups and work primarily to deregulate environmental regulations. Labor groups are often recruited to narrate a story of job creation to justify environmentally damaging projects framed as development in spite of the evidence that the numbers of local jobs created by these projects are fairly limited. Academics, as experts paid for by the structures of neoliberal instrumentality, serve as the uncritical mouthpieces for these TNCs, with mainstream media working hand in hand to circulate the TNC discourses, recruiting many of these academics as pundits on 24-7 news cycles.

Communicative inversions cast as outside the realm of the "acceptable" questions regarding conflicts of interests, private funding of science, biases introduced into scientific representation by the injection of private money into science, and the revolving door among academia, industry, think tanks, lobbies, government, and regulatory bodies. Health privatizing management organizations, for instance, invert their profiteering agendas in a narrative of delivering health access and efficient health care. The narrative of building efficient systems circulates a story of weak governance and dissipation of resources in state bureaucracies while at the same time erasing questions of profit-making motives, managerial salaries, and effectiveness of access directed at the for-profit structures. Communicative inversions are primarily carried out through public relations and advertising activities. Through these communicative inversions, neoliberalism offers an image of dialogue and consultation, portraying a facade of listening even as neoliberal communication solutions utilize dialogue and listening instrumentally to achieve predetermined objectives and goals.

The work of communication is closely tied to achieving communicative inversions and communicative erasures, systematically producing knowledge structures that reify the organizing logics of neoliberalism. In his *For a New Critique of Political Economy*, Bernard Steigler (2009) discusses the "proletarianization of the nervous system," marked by the hegemony of cognitive technologies that have been reduced to technologies of calculability. Referring to this routinization of knowledge-producing processes within technological rationalities of neoliberalism as "cognitive capitalism," Steigler (2009) observes:

> If skilled professions [métiers] do in fact still remain, very few are connected with that type of production that is called "creative," and most of the time such jobs are not really creative. For to be creative—that is, to work [*oeuvrer*—to work on something, to open up a work]—is to produce negentropy. But those who are called "creative workers" today are in fact merely creators of that kind of "value" which is *capable of being evaluated on the market,* like press officers or public relations officials who work toward the *entropic adaptation* of the system, but who do not create any works or open up any work. (pp. 45–46)

The work of communication thus is routinized into the structures of neoliberalism, performing the everyday erasures and inversions that leave intact the structures of neoliberal governance across global spaces, albeit taking different forms within different local systems and simultaneously fostering global networks of communicative spaces that exert the hegemony of the neoliberal organizing order. Events management, press relations, publicity, crisis management, and other forms of communication activities are constituted within the parameters of recycling the consumerist, short-term, and individualist logics of neoliberalism. Communication thus gets constrained in its creative ability to imagine alternative forms of organizing. The next section engages with these creative possibilities of communication.

Imagination, Creativity, and Alternative Organizing

This book set out to examine closely the dominant interpretations of health, healing, and curing reproduced within neoliberal structures of health organizing. I hope that this last section of the book serves as an invitation for imaginations, working through articulations of various transformative possibilities that are being opened up by communities across the globe, working in spaces of solidarity in reshaping the health narrative in resistance to the very limited and limiting neoliberal story. The limited and culturally particular formulation of the neoliberal model of health derived from Northern/Western models of linear development situated within white liberal imaginations of health and well-being are being disrupted actively by subaltern voices emerging from the global South that are actively working in collectives and in collaborative communities.

Drawing from the interconnected layers of critical thought that emerge from postcolonial and subaltern studies theories into the ambits of the social scientific work of social change and health communication, the culture-centered approach offers an invitation into solidarity with subaltern communities at the global margins that actively participate every day in offering creative visions of collective ownership, community collaborations, and community-driven networks of social change. For many of these communities, the bourgeoisie notion of social change that has been co-opted into the academic–civil society–corporate–state structures is the very site of intervention, connecting social change to processes of structural transformation that begin with the acknowledgment that neoliberalism is a faulty and health threatening organizational structure that needs to be systematically undone in order to promote spaces of health and well-being.

Challenging the neoliberal vision of participation as an instrument for disseminating dominant agendas configured by IFIs preaching a narrowly West-centric model of development predicated on the hegemony of the free market, culturally centered processes of social change from the global margins depict the role of participation as an entry point for accountability to local community visions, local community understanding of problems, and the imagination of solutions embedded within community interpretations. The state thus, as a resource and as a structure of governance, is rendered accountable to the local community, structurally transformed through local participatory processes toward addressing community needs. Local participation interprets state policies within the context of the organic contexts of local communities.

Knowledge, articulated in conversations and dialogues within local communities, in organic community linkages and democratic ties, resists the dominant structures of neoliberal knowledge that are implicitly tied to agendas of profiteering and free market capitalism. That capitalism is not intrinsic to ideas and aspirations of democracy is a key strand that is continually articulated in subaltern social movements across the global South. That the ideas of democracy and democratic participation need to be fundamentally decoupled from the rhetoric of the free market, market-driven liberty, and individually-driven selfish participation is being voiced by subaltern communities resisting privatization, displacement, and the heuristic of growth-driven development. That growth itself is not always a good thing, but rather needs to be understood in relationship to power and distributions of resources and needs to be examined in relationship to the toxic health effects of an unchecked growth narrative is an idea that is emerging from across subaltern communities in the global South. Subaltern social movements against mining, urbanization, displacement, dams, worker vulnerability, worker exploitation, privatization of nature, and corporatization of agriculture are some examples of the emerging subaltern voices from across the globe. The notion of democracy in organic interstices of community ties and community participatory processes is actively being reworked in resistance to the monolithic construction of functional communities as instruments of message dissemination and propaganda in top-down WB-led interventions. Communication is actively being reimagined spatially, as a site for fostering alternative spaces of articulation and as a constitutive framework for imaginations.

New World Information Communication Order (NWICO)

One example of the active reworking of communicative spaces is NWICO. The NWICO was envisioned by UNESCO as a space for fostering communicative equalities by directly opposing the current framework of unequal organizing of media spaces dominated by Western media organizations and transnational capital. The imaginations of the NWICO, in other words, were rooted in aspirations for communicative spaces that fostered sovereignty and participation of the grass roots, actively engaging with possibilities of creating alternative structures of communication. The NWICO threatened the U.S. imperial control of large media structures that works in nexus with transnational hegemony, and thus was actively opposed by the U.S.-transnational capital nexus (Nordenstreng, 2012; Pickard, 2007). Integral to the articulation of the NWICO was an emphasis placed on fostering opportunities for communication across global spaces, attending to the inequalities in media and technology ownership patterns, and suggesting pathways for addressing these inequalities.

Challenging the inequities in health requires a fundamental interrogation of the "free market" model of media policies and global media governance, interrogating the health consequences of the global hegemony of privatized Western media and exploring possibilities for listening to local meanings of health and well-being rooted in the lived experiences of local communities at the global margins. Inviting opportunities for other imaginations is intertwined with the struggles of social justice that are directed at fostering spaces for participation and communication, rooted in the struggles for health and well-being in subaltern communities amid neoliberal reforms that threaten human health. As opposed to the top-down techno-deterministic framework of creating the next "app" to enable equality or community participation or individual lifestyle change, technology is intertwined with community processes and spaces of transformation directed at addressing the unequal structures that shape health outcomes. The role of communication is transformed from one of designing culturally sensitive health promotion messages directed at marginalized communities (Bresnahan et al., 2007; Kreuter et al., 2013) to fostering local community spaces for participation, articulation, and information sharing, connected to national and global networks and creating entry points for sharing diverse understandings of health and well-being. Communicative spaces of accountability co-created within local, global, and national structures offer opportunities for holding state, market, and civil society actors accountable to local community voices. Thomas (2011) for instance discusses the example of the *Jan Sunwais* in India, local meetings presided over by a panel of respected individuals in the local community, that hold development actors accountable through public meetings where specific charges of corruption on development projects are brought up by community members on the basis of extensive research conducted by volunteers, and development actors are given an opportunity to clarify the accounts, project deliverables, and project details. The public hearing is organized independently and is widely publicized among villagers. Government officials, elected representatives and the press are invited to the hearings. Official records of amounts sanctioned and actually spent on local development projects are obtained from local government offices. Various stakeholders working on the development project are offered opportunities for providing their accounts of work done, salaries received, etc. In an excerpt from the *Lokniti* Newsletter (2005), Thomas (2011, p. 102) points to the important role of voice:

> . . . an empowering process in that, it not only does away with civil society structures that are stacked against the marginalized but also inverts power equations in favour of the marginalized, by making them the centre of the discussion. There are no experts and "hence no chance of objectification of the victim" and the "victim represents his case without any technical assistance."

In similar grounded citizens' juries for health activism carried out in the north-east of England, local community participation formed on the basis of deliberation, integration, sustainability and accountability led to the setting up of a community health center (Kashefi & Mort, 2004). Participation was thus reconfigured in the context of a local jury weighing evidence to make the most meaningful health decisions, resisting the mechanical function of participation in top-down consultative processes in neoliberal structures. Along similar lines, voice emerges as the heart of the Occupy movement, seeking to foster symbolic spaces for transforming neoliberal economic policies that threaten human health and well-being (Dutta, 2013).

The emphasis therefore is on fostering communicative capacities for articulating local meanings of health and well-being, and aligning these meanings with local access to health promoting resources grounded in the aspirations of local communities. For instance, creating spaces across the global margins for resisting the commoditization of medicine and the privatization of knowledge under the ambits of trade-related intellectual property rights (TRIPS) fosters possibilities for creating access to medicines among the poor (Subramanian, 1994). Doing so also calls for creating and fostering avenues for communication that bypass the silences and biases produced by corporate-owned media that draw their revenues from advertising (such as advertising from pharmaceutical corporations). Similarly, resisting the neoliberal structures of biopiracy at the intersections of research centers, universities, and transnational corporations creates entry points for regaining the sovereignty of local communities over healing resources indigenous to these communities (Shiva, 2001, 2007, 2010). Access to spaces of articulation is fundamental to establishing claims on knowledge grounded in local culture and local frameworks of meaning. Everyday spaces of communication as well as communication technologies in the mainstream are mobilized for the purposes of generating alternative articulations of health and well-being. Digital and new media platforms that serve as instruments of neoliberal control are co-opted into the struggles of resistance in subaltern communities, in building global network capacities locally, in creating global networks of resistance connected to local voices of resistance, and in challenging neoliberal hegemony at the centers of global capitalism through the voicing of local interpretations. In the resistance of the *Dongria Kondh* to the *Vedanta* mining operations that threatened their livelihood, health, and well-being, local participation in processes of change was complemented with solidarity networks of activism connected through the online platform *Foil Vedanta* and staging protests at the financial center of *Vedanta* in London (Dutta, 2013). The resistance voiced by women farmers in Andhra Pradesh organized under the ambits of the *Deccan Development Society* is organized through community radio that is owned and run by the women farmers (Pavarala & Malik, 2007). Communicative equality, depicted in the form of creating communicative spaces that are authentic to local participation and local voices, is intertwined with organizing processes directed at bringing economic equality and equality in access to juridical spaces for holding TNCs accountable. The struggles for health and for addressing health disparities are therefore not simply about promoting healthy lifestyles and health-based knowledge, but are integral to participatory processes seeking transformations in the very structures of neoliberal hegemony that threaten human health and well-being. At a global level, such invitations for fostering communicative equalities seek to invert the unequal terrains of power that constitute the discursive sphere of communication, fundamentally thus reconfiguring the meaning of communication and the relationship of communication to structures of organizing.

Social Medicine

Latin American social medicine depicts a distinct and long strand of theorizing of health systems that challenges the liberal capitalist organizing of health, grounded in the organizing principles of social medicine and noting that changing the overarching structures is central to transforming the conditions of poor health (Waitzkin, 1991, 2011; Waitzkin & Modell, 1974). That health is constituted within broader social conditions is the basis for research, teaching, clinical practice, and activism in socialist medicine, with early roots in Latin America. Social medicine thus connects health, healing, and health care delivery to the politics of social change and structural transformation, clearly voicing an activist agenda directed at transforming the unequal social conditions.

One of the earliest influences of social medicine was evident in the work of the medical student activist Salvador Allende, who would later become the president of Chile. In his book *The Chilean Medico-Social Reality*, Allende (1939) outlined the social conditions in Chile that resulted in poor health outcomes, emphasizing the broader conditions of foreign debt dependence, underdevelopment, international dependence, and resource consolidation in the hands of the local elite. Proposing social rather than medical solutions to health, Allende emphasized "income redistribution, state regulation of food and clothing supplies, a national housing program, and industrial reforms to address occupational health problems" (Waitzkin, 2011, p. 160). In his political life, Allende sought reforms in the Chilean national health service, complemented by reforms in the housing and nutrition areas, efforts at national income redistribution, and minimizing the role of multinational corporations.

The individualized model of public health that sees health and illness as a dichotomy is interrogated by the framework of social medicine that suggests that health and illness exist in a dialectical relationship that is dynamic and is continually shifting on the basis of social conditions, structures, cultural practices, economic production, reproduction, marginalizing practices, and processes of political participation. Thus, interventions in social medicine point toward the necessity for transforming the underlying relationships of production and resource distribution, resisting the public health narrative of interventions as mechanisms for improving economic productivity. Taking a social-class-driven approach to health inequities, Latin American social medicine sees the problems with health being situated within means of economic production, patterns of ownership of means of production, and control over productive processes. Therefore, health is approached from the framework of transforming the processes of economic production and labor processes.

The dominant framework of health as integral to growth and economic productivity is questioned by the framework of social medicine that situates the relationship between health and illness amid the very processes of economic organization, distribution of economic resources, and the pervasive effects of social class on health services and health outcomes.

The innovations in organizing of health structures in Chile, Cuba, Mexico, Bolivia, and Venezuela offer invaluable insights about the possibilities of alternative organizing that seek to redo the entire structure of social organizing that constitute health. The strong health indicators in Cuba demonstrate the effectiveness of a health system that is committed to addressing the structural determinants of health, creating equitable contexts for the realization and delivery of health (Campion & Morrissey, 2013). Social medicine research has looked at the relations among work, reproduction, the environment, and health, describing in-depth the material conditions that constitute health. For instance, researchers studying health in Mexico within the context of unions and local communities have documented health problems that relate to work processes and the environment. Similarly, researchers in Chile have documented the relations between gender, work, and environmental conditions. A key strand of social medicine examines the relationship between violence and health, connecting violence to poverty, the structures of organizing, and the inequities in ownership of processes of economic production. Investigations of violence attached to the U.S.-supported dictatorship in Chile, the violence connected to narcotics traffic and paramilitary operations, and the violence within the broader structures of the state-imperial networks draw linkages to the broader political economic configurations of neoliberalism.

Emerging from the broader framework of social medicine, the *Barrio Adentro* movement in Venezuela, started by former president Hugo Chavez, offers insights into structures and processes of alternative organizing of health, connecting local community structures, community ownership, and community solutions with state infrastructures and state-driven public health resources and solutions (Briggs & Mantini-Briggs, 2009; Muntaner et al., 2006; Waitzkin, 2011). The state-driven referendum by the Chavez government to create public health infrastructures and structures of delivery of integrated family medicine, build preventive infrastructures, and develop community health resources in extremely marginalized communities is supported by massive mass-based participation in popular politics and widespread community participation in developing local community infrastructures, community-based resources of problem solving, and community decision-making capacities. The community health centers built within the barrios serve approximately 250 families and are staffed with one integrated family care doctor, one community health worker, and one health promoter. The community health centers are stocked with medical supplies. The health team not only provides health care but also conducts health surveys in the communities and makes home visits for patients that are too ill to travel to the health centers. The *Barrio Adentro* is integrated with other *missiones* addressing education, food insecurity, housing, and unemployment, addressing health within a broader structural context (Muntaner et al., 2006). Local community participatory processes are connected with state-driven processes of building community health infrastructures at the local level.

The narrative of *Barrio Adentro* offers an alternative to the neoliberal narrative of the community in mainstream health communication and yet is marked by its absence from disciplinary discourses. Similarly, social medicine and its tradition of addressing the structural contexts of health is marked by its absence from the dominant discourses of health communication. A review of the two major collections of health communication scholarship, *The Routledge Handbook of Health Communication* and *The Handbook of Global Health Communication*, depicts the marked absence of the Latin American innovations of social medicine from the discursive space. Opportunities for resistance to neoliberal organizing of health structures and the invitation to imagine alternative possibilities is grounded in materially grounded concrete politics of popular participation in supporting state policies for building public health and health care infrastructures, complemented by local processes of participation in the creation of health solutions.

Alternative Forms and Processes of Organizing

Listening to communities at the global margins brings forth narratives of organizing that are grounded in understandings of human health and human relationships that challenge the psychologized model of health organizing rooted in the atomized individual. Narratives of cooperation and collective ownership, for instance, challenge the individualized model of health organizing. Narratives of living in harmony with nature interrogate the normalized narratives of controlling nature. The locus of responsibility is shifted from the self-caring individual with motivation and ability to collective networks of care and ownership, collectively articulating notions of sustainability, harmonious relationship with the environment, and cooperative processes of participation. Opening up conversations about alternative forms and processes of organizing fosters new spaces for global solidarities in South–South networks.

In the example of the *Barrio Adentro* initiative discussed above, the role played by Cuban doctors in responding to a call issued by President Chavez of Venezuela for integrated family physicians under the Cuban government's international solidarity program depict the possibilities of global South–South solidarity that bypass the imperial, profit-driven structures of international health assistance offered under the rubrics of the IFIs. Similarly, the recent role played by Cuban doctors in responding to the Ebola epidemic in Western Africa depicts another example of South to South collaboration and solidarity. Within the broader politics of global health, these South–South networks of collaboration and support offer alternative entry points for imagining health as a fundamental human right constituted in a structure of equal and open access, realized through democratic participation.

Also, local organizing for health seeks to transform the underlying causes of poor health within community spaces. For instance, community-driven zoning projects seeking to regulate the number of fast food restaurants in the community are driven by an emphasis on intervening in policy structures. Such interventions to regulate the flow of unhealthy products are carried out at local, regional, national, and global levels, often depicting strategies of solidarity across local levels networked into national and global level spaces of resistance. The popular participation movements across India catalyze the participatory capacity of local communities to articulate criteria for accountability and transparency directed at political and economic policies. Grassroots participatory processes in the realm of the local resist the co-optation of mainstream media to sell the neoliberal agendas of transnational hegemony. Door to door participation in everyday politics among the subaltern classes disrupts the lobby-driven economically formulated version of politics. The hegemonic mainstream media framework promoting the neoliberal logic is disrupted by grassroots-level participation.

Interventions in media structures seek to regulate the advertising of harmful fast food and sugary drinks/colas directed at children across global spaces. Efforts of regulating tobacco advertising are carried out in local-national-global networks, with knowledge being shared across spaces to develop effective strategies for resisting the power exerted by the fast food industry or the tobacco industry (Yach, Wipfli, Hammond & Glantz, 2008). Articulations of media regulation anchored in claims to health are juxtaposed against neoliberal articulations of free trade across global borders. Thus, communication and media themselves emerge as sites of contestation in organizing for health. The counterhegemonic power exerted over mainstream media by subaltern movements, popular movements, and grassroots processes of social change offer opportunities for rendering transparent the hidden linkages between powerful economic and political forces that threaten human health and well-being. For instance, multiple news channels joined in solidarity in depicting the ways in which HSBC worked to hide the tax evasion funds of the global elite, instructing the elite on strategies for tax evasion through the strategic use of offshore accounts (Leigh et al., 2015). Similarly, the role of HSBC in funding arms dealers and drug cartels becomes evident in the investigative work titled “Swiss Leaks” carried out by the International Consortium of Investigative Journalists (ICIJ, 2015).

Reimagining Civil Society in Resistive Processes

Just as civil society has been historically interjected into the structures of global neoliberal control driven by the politics of donor funding and the rhetoric of empowerment (Barker, M. J., 2004), examples of civil society–activist–community partnerships in the global South point toward alternative possibilities for the organizing of civil societies that are driven by community voices and community participation in everyday processes of social change (Dutta, 2011, 2013). As is elucidated through the community participatory processes in the *Niyamgiri* movement led by the *Dongria Kondh* residing in the Niyamgiri Hills, processes of participation and collaboration with activist communities and with NGOs fosters opportunities in subaltern communities for circulating the message of social change globally (Padel & Das, 2010). The interpretations of health and well-being in the life-world of the community become catalytic agents for connecting global struggles for social change (Dutta, 2013). Moreover, locally situated movements such as the *Niyamgiri* movement also become points of inspiration for other similar movements, offering communicative entry points and frameworks of resistance to the logics of neoliberal development. For instance, voicing of the threats to health posed by the mining operations in Niyamgiri emerge as anchors for similar articulations of threats to health in subaltern struggles against displacement by mining (Dutta, 2013; Padel & Das, 2010). Struggles against the exploitation of Ogoniland in Nigeria and the voicing of threats to health posed by oil drilling operations carried out by the collusion of Shell and the Nigerian state emerge as exemplars for global struggles against threats to health posed by neoliberal models of oil and mineral extraction (Dutta, 2011; Obi, 1997). Resistance against the privatization of water in Cochabamba emerges as an exemplar of transformative social change processes articulating the notion of health in the context of the commons and public resources (Olivera & Lewis, 2004).

Entry points into the dominant structures of civil society are fostered through processes of activist–community–civil society collaborations initiated by subaltern communities. Subaltern rationalities enter into the realms of contestation and claims making within neoliberal structures. Legal cases on biopiracy, for instance, fought by teams of lawyers, activists, and subaltern communities from the global South interrupt the strategies of theft and colonialism written into the structures of neoliberalism and justified as patents. For instance, the patenting of Basmati by U.S.-based RiceTec was fought in global courts by teams of lawyers, state representatives, and activists representing subaltern claims on indigenous knowledge through parallel conversations in subaltern contexts and in dominant elite-controlled structures of neoliberal globalization (Dutta, 2011; Dutta & Pal, 2010).

The realm of accountability, the scope of decision making, and the range of problems and solutions are all developed by community members who have historically been erased. Entry points into juridical structures that are otherwise owned and controlled by dominant social actors with specific forms of access to the formalized and specialized language of law are secured through civil society–activist–community linkages. Lawyers working in solidarity with communities in processes of social change from below transform the neoliberal claims to consolidation of resources in the hands of the global elite through appeals to laws voicing claims of subaltern communities. These processes of participation in resisting neoliberal structures through juridical processes is complemented by popular politics, politics of participation in protests, and globally linked protests at sites of neoliberal enunciations such as protests at board member meetings of TNCs, protests at annual stakeholder meetings of TNCs, and campaigns directed at shareholders and investment portfolios.

Role of the State and Popular Politics

The state, in the subaltern spheres of participation, is closely tied to subaltern aspirations expressed through participation in everyday politics (Chatterjee, 2004). Subaltern communities, often having been erased from the dominant discursive spaces reflected by civil society organizations in the mainstream, participate in the politics of the everyday to secure access to the very resources that are often usurped by these powerful civil society organizations in service of the elite classes. Having been erased from the structures of civil society by the very languages and tools required for participation in the civil society, subaltern communities forge their realms of everyday participation in securing resources from the state (Dutta, 2013b). The arena of political society emerges as a site of active contestation and resistance, leveraging the everyday networks of political power to secure resources for the community, and enacting various forms of agency through a wide array of communication channels to resist the consolidation of power in the hands of local-national-global elites. The participation of subaltern communities in processes of resistance is often directed at strengthening state-based public provisions and the delivery of public goods, seeking to hold the mechanisms of delivery and distribution of public resources accountable to participatory processes that are grounded in local communities, experiences of community members, and community voices. Community-driven participatory processes in social change demand transparency and accountability from the powerful stakeholders at various levels, holding civil society, development, and political actors accountable to grassroots democracy. Forms of communication beyond the mainstream media such as street art, songs, dances, street theater, public protests, and public performances are catalyzed as resources for narrating stories of resistance (Dutta, 2013b).

Openings for alternative imaginations of local–global organizing of health emerge from the spaces of political society, depicting the very creative and innovative processes through which health rights are secured and fought for by the subaltern classes who are otherwise erased from elite discursive spheres of decision making. Alternative forms of organizing such as collectives and cooperatives offer alternative entry points for imagining communication for health. As in the example of Venezuela, popular support for health structures driven by a framework of universal access inspires the political legitimacy for alternative organizing. Popular support through political processes also resists the co-optation strategies and resource consolidation strategies deployed by the middle and upper-middle classes with the agenda of personal profiteering. Subaltern participation in politics thus works in the backdrop of neoliberalism as a legitimate entry point for articulating alternative values and visions, exerting pressure on states and policymakers and resisting the pressures exerted by TNCs through lobbies, political donations, and public relations exercises. Open and popular participation in democratic processes at the grassroots level resist the opaque processes of resource consolidation in the hands of the transnational elite. Participation thus is reconfigured from being an instrument of neoliberal expansion to an ingredient in the democratic process of grassroots decision making, working with state structures to strengthen them, working with civil society to foster new entry points for accountability, and holding the market accountability to local community voices.

Resisting Reductionism and toward Integration

As noted throughout the book, the power of neoliberal interventions globally is constituted on the basis of the reductionist logic of narrowing down on the individual, and subsequently on a specific body part as the site of empowerment/intervention. The empowerment/intervention inversion is integral to neoliberal processes where the intervention framed as individual empowerment in enactment of choices as a consumer works alongside the depletion of public health infrastructures, the large-scale reproduction of inequalities and health disparities by unequal structures of political and economic organizing, and the profits generated by the privatization of health across the globe. Promoting exercising, for instance, becomes an entire cottage industry of its own, generating new markets for apps, measurement devices, reality shows, and message-tailoring platforms. Significant resources are expended on individualized solutions such as promoting the consumption of fruits and vegetables, while at the same time obfuscating the large-scale corporatization of food resources and the consolidation of food/agriculture as a site of transnational profiteering. Pharmaceutical solutions prescribing individualized remedies of self-improvement offer new markets for global profiteering, creating new conditions that call for new pharmaceutical commodities to be marketed and simultaneously obfuscating the broader structural threats to human health and well-being.

This reductionist approach to biomedicine translates into an overarching reductionist framework of health communication, with health communication solutions focusing on a specific disease state or on promoting a specific behavior without placing the illness and behavior within the broader societal context. Structures, social contexts, and the unequal patterns of resource distribution in societies are erased from the discursive space. For instance, in discussions of cancer inequalities, interventions often solely focus on promoting individual behaviors, oblivious to the structural and environmental contexts of cancer risks. Even when structures are mentioned in a cursory footnote or conclusion section, such as in the realm of the growing body of health disparities research, the solutions proposed are often focused on the individual, without really developing avenues for addressing the structures or without really creating pathways for transforming them. Culture is used as a tool for developing culturally sensitive campaigns that measure cultural characteristics to develop more effective and efficient solutions that would address the cultural values that act as barriers. Culture is individualized as a receptacle of backward values that get in the way of the individual adoption of the promoted behavior. The deficit model that places culture in the role of an impediment therefore seeks to generate culturally sensitive messages that take cultural characteristics into account to deliver more effective health messages.

The language of culture, communication, and change embody neoliberal violence where the blame, once placed on the culture, emerges as a leveraging tool for white liberal solutions to cultural deficits. In the context of heart disease for instance, the emphasis is placed on lifestyle choices without attending to the availability of food or the availability of pathways for exercising. Structural features such as inaccess to basic health and lack of education and economic opportunities in African American communities in the United States, the history of racism in the United States, the absence of health infrastructures, food deserts in African American communities, and the lack of economic opportunities experienced by African Americans in the United States are erased from the discursive space. That poverty offers a vital context for understanding meanings of health is undermined and obfuscated, categorically marked as the outside of what counts as mainstream health communication and delineating the scope of health communication as the development of messages targeting individual behavior change.

Within neoliberal structures that constitute the language and terminologies of the field, knowledge production processes work actively to establish the hegemony of the message-centric approach, defining legitimacy narrowly in the ambits of health communication as message testing and message production. What counts as acceptable health communication scholarship is defined narrowly within the ambits of the Cold War history of the discipline, placing emphasis on communication as a vehicle of persuasion and strategic conversion. The functionalism of health communication in the prevailing discourse is attached thus to the reproduction of the dominant structures. For instance, the persuasion literature in health campaigns inadvertently targets individual beliefs, attitudes, and behaviors, and not the broader structural contexts of health. For instance, we don't witness health communication scholarship that is targeted at persuading individuals to support public policies of universal and equal access to health care. Questions of power, meaning, inequality, political and economic organizing, social processes of organization, racist structures of meaning construction, and so on, remain erased from the discursive spaces of what counts as mainstream communication and health. The definition of communication as messages obfuscates the possibilities of understanding health communication as meanings, interpretations, and negotiations, constituted in relationship to structures of power, inequality, and differential access to health resources.

The culture-centered approach is positioned in resistance to these traditional structures of health communication, interrogating the limits of the individual-based model and seeking spaces for integrating experiences, of connecting the dots, and of developing integrative narratives that examine health as constituted through language. The possibilities of resistance are thus marked in the openings offered through the interrogation and theorizing of structures. That knowledge production itself is a political process established through communication depicts the centrality of communication as a theoretical lens. The attention placed on meanings and interpretations situated in relationship to power and control offers openings for understanding the ways in which dominant structures actively construct meanings of health, what these structures erase in these constructions, and the kinds of agendas that are accomplished through these acts of erasure. Close reading of what makes up common sense also serves as a strategy for developing fluid, interactive, and integrative solution frameworks that attend to the interplays of the individual, the relational, the family, the community, and the broader society. Listening emerges in this backdrop as a strategy for centering the voices of communities that have hitherto been erased. Structural transformations are introduced as agendas for health communication scholarship, working in solidarity with subaltern communities.

Conclusion

The recent Ebola outbreaks in West Africa narrate the fault lines of neoliberal health organizing, constituted in the dramatic inequalities, inequalities in distribution of resources, and the weakening of public health systems, services, and infrastructures especially in the marginalized sectors of the globe (WHO, 2014). The dilapidation of health systems, weakening of public health infrastructures, and the inequalities in the distribution of infrastructures of care brought about by neoliberal reforms become evident in the patterns of distribution of the disease, the high mortality rates in resource-poor areas, and the absence of adequate health care to offer healing to patients. The WHO report on Ebola also depicts the paradoxes of thinking wrapped up in an overarching neoliberal frame as in spite of its reference to growing inequalities and poor public health systems, the WHO report diagnoses solutions in the language of economic losses. These paradoxes and communicative inversions are integral to the structures of neoliberal organizing, suggesting an important role for health communicators in interrogating closely the meaning structures and interpretive frameworks circulated in mainstream discourses of health. Spaces of imaginations and alternative rationalities need to be actively fostered in offering new ways of addressing health at the margins of neoliberal globalization. These alternative rationalities suggest the necessity for understanding health not as an isolated entity, but as intertwined with societal, cultural, political, and economic processes. The possibilities of health organizing thus are rooted in active imaginations of alternative economic and political structures that interrogate the values of selfishness, greed, consumption, and commoditization brought about by the global diffusion of neoliberalism through a variety of development projects.

Voices from the global margins put forth frameworks of health and healing that interrogate the linear trajectories of development circulated in Western/white liberalism based on binaries driven by heuristics of consumption, market, technological fixes, and reductionist thinking. In wrapping up, this book reviewed the key arguments in the mainstream structures of neoliberal health organizing, attending to the taken-for-granted meanings that form the foundations for neoliberal ideas. Close reading of these structures depicts the interplays between IFIs, state, NGOs, and TNCs. The individualization of health, the deployment of behavioral and lifestyle solutions, and the erasure of structures are part of the neoliberal plot.

Resisting the neoliberal plot therefore is tied to an active search for other imaginations, grounded in alternative visions of the good life and meanings of well-being. Narratives of cooperation, organic relationships with communities of care, a harmonious relationship with nature, and dialogues rooted in difference offer new entry points for working on possibilities of social change and structural transformation. The specificities of local organizing rooted in notions of difference and cultural situatedness offer new frameworks for global learning guided by creative interpretations and organizing processes at the local level. It is my hope that this series in Critical Cultural Studies in Global Health Communication will offer tentative entry points for reimagining questions of human health and well-being, centering the study and practice of health communication as explorations of interpretations and narratives that are situated within negotiations and contestations of power and that are integral to the quest for a just and healthy global society.

REFERENCES

Aaltola, M. (2012). Contagious insecurity: War, SARS and global air mobility. *Contemporary Politics, 18*(1), 53–70.

Adeleye, O. A., Aldoory, L., & Parakoyi, D. B. (2011). Using local culture and gender roles to improve male involvement in maternal health in southern Nigeria. *Journal of Health Communication, 16*(10), 1122–1135.

AFDR. (2000). *Suicides in rural area of Punjab: A report (in Punjabi).* Ludhiana: Association for Democratic Rights.

Allende, S. (1939). *La realidad medico-social Chilena.* Santiago, Chile: Ministerio de Salubridad.

Alliance for Human Research Protection. (2011). Report blasts unethical HPV vaccine trial in India. Retrieved from www.ahrp.org/cms/content/view/805/52/ on June 5, 2014.

Amin, A. (1997). Placing globalization. *Theory, Culture & Society, 14*(2), 123–137.

Appadurai, A. (2011). Disjuncture and difference in the global cultural economy 1990. *Theory, Culture, & Society, 7,* 295–310.

Armada, F., Muntaner, C., & Navarro, V. (2001). Health and social security reforms in Latin America: The convergence of the World Health Organization, the World Bank, and transnational corporations. *International Journal of Health Services, 31,* 729–768.

Armand, F., O'Hanlon, B., McEuen, M., Kolyada, L., and Levin, L. (2007). *Private sector contribution to family planning and contraceptive security in the Europe and Eurasia region.* Bethesda, MD: Private Sector Partnerships-One project, Abt Associates.

Artz, L. (2006). On the material and the dialectic: Toward a class analysis of communication. In L. Artz, S. Macek, & D. Cloud (Eds.), *Marxism and communication studies: The point is to change it* (pp. 5–51). New York: Peter Lang.

Avahan—The India AIDS Initiative (2008). The business of HIV prevention at scale. Paper prepared for the Bill & Melinda Gates Foundation. New Delhi: Bill & Melinda Gates Foundation.

Baglia, J. (2005). *The Viagra ad venture: Masculinity, media, and the performance of sexual health.* New York: Peter Lang.

Barker, K. (2004). Diffusion of innovations: A world tour. *Journal of Health Communication, 9,* 131–137.

Barker, M. J. (2004). *Civil society, empowered or overpowered: The role of the mass media in "promoting democracy" worldwide.* Retrieved from www.adelaide.edu.au/anzca2006/conf_proceedings/barker_mj_civilsociety_empowered_overpowered.pdf on August 11, 2014.

Becker, J., & Van Natta, D. (2008). After mining deal, financier donated to Clinton. *New York Times,* January 31, A1.

Berman, R. (2014). The US military wages war on Ebola. *Atlantic*, October 7. Retrieved from www.theatlantic.com/national/archive/2014/10/the-us-military-wages-war-on-ebola/381197/ on October 9, 2014.

Bertrand, J. T., Babalola, S., & Skinner, J. (2012). The impact of health communication programs. In R. Obregon & S. Waisbord (Eds.), *The Handbook of Global Health Communication* (pp. 97–120). Malden, MA: Wiley-Blackwell.

Bodekar, G. (2003). Traditional medicine knowledge, intellectual property rights & benefit sharing. *Cardozo Journal of International & Comparitive Law*, 11: 785–814.

Booth, R. (2013). Qatar World Cup construction 'will leave 4,000 migrant workers dead.' *Guardian*. Retrieved from www.theguardian.com/global-development/2013/sep/26/qatar-world-cup-migrant-workers-dead on February 24, 2015.

Boulay, M., & Valente, T. (2005). The selection of family planning discussion partners in Nepal. *Journal of Health Communication, 10*, 519–536.

Bourdieu, P. (1998). The essence of neoliberalism. *Le Monde Diplomatique*, December 8. Retrieved from mondediplo.com/1998/12/08boudieu on January 10, 2014.

Brenner, J., Ross, J., Simmons, J., & Zaidi, S. (2000). Neoliberal trade and investment and the health of Maquiladora workers on the U.S.-Mexico border. In J. Y. Kim, J. V. Millen, A. Irwin, & J. Gershman (Eds.), *Dying for growth: Global inequality and the health of the poor* (pp. 261–290). Monroe, ME: Common Courage Press.

Bresnahan, M., Lee, S. Y., Smith, S. W., Shearman, S., Nebashi, R., Park, C. Y., & Yoo, J. (2007). A theory of planned behavior study of college students' intention to register as organ donors in Japan, Korea, and the United States. *Health Communication, 21*(3), 201–211.

Briggs, C. L., & Mantini-Briggs, C. (2009). Confronting health disparities: Latin American social medicine in Venezuela. *American Journal of Public Health, 99*(3), 549.

Brossard, D., Shanahan, J., & Nesbitt, T. C. (2007). *The media, the public and agricultural biotechnology*. Oxon, UK: CABI.

Brown, B. J., & Baker, S. (2012). *Responsible citizens: Individuals, health and policy under neoliberalism*. London: Anthem Press.

Buley, T. (2010). Start-up goes public on Corbis fraud, starring Bill Gates. *Forbes.com*, July 19. Retrieved from www.forbes.com/2010/07/19/corbis-infoflows-lawsuit-technology-bill-gates.html?boxes=techchanneltopstories on August 28, 2014.

Burton, B. (2007). *Inside spin: The dark underbelly of the PR industry*. Crows Nest, Australia: Allen & Unwin.

Buse, K., & Waxman, A. (2001). Public–private health partnerships: A strategy for WHO. *Bulletin of the World Health Organization, 79*, 748–754.

Bush, G. W. (2002). *Biodefense for the 21st century*. Washington, DC: White House.

Caballero, M. (2005). SARS in Asia: Crisis, vulnerabilities and regional responses. *Asian Survey, 45*(3), 475–495.

Caballero-Anthony, M. (2006). Combating infectious diseases in East Asia: Securitization and global public goods for health and human security. *Journal of International Affairs, 59*(2), 105.

Caduff, C. (2010). Public prophylaxis: Pandemic influenza, pharmaceutical prevention and participatory governance. *BioSocieties, 5*(2), 199–218.

Campbell, H. C. (2014). Understanding the US policy of diplomacy, development, and defense: The Office of Transition Initiatives and the Subversion of Societies. *CounterPunch*. Retrieved from www.counterpunch.org/2014/05/02/the-office-of-transition-initiatives-and-the-subversion-of-societies/ on February 22, 2015.

Campbell, J. L., & Peterson, O. K. (2001). *The rise of neoliberalism and institutional analysis*. Princeton, NJ: Princeton University Press.

Campion, E. W., & Morrissey, S. (2013). A different model—Medical care in Cuba. *New England Journal of Medicine, 368*(4), 297–299.

Carmichael, A. G. (1986). *Plague and the poor in renaissance Florence*. Cambridge: Cambridge University Press.

Carroll, W., & Carson, C. (2006). Neoliberalism, capitalist class formation and the global network of corporations and policy groups. In D. Plewhe, B. Walpen, & G. Nuenhoffer (Eds.), *Neoliberal hegemony: A global critique* (pp. 42–73). London: Routledge.

Chan, J., & Ngai, P. (2010). Suicide as protest for the new generation of Chinese migrant workers: Foxconn, global capital, and the state. *Asia-Pacific Journal: Japan Focus, 37*(2). Retrieved from www.japanfocus.org/-Jenny-Chan/3408 on May 15, 2014.

Chandrasekhar, C. P., & Ghosh, J. (2001). Information and communication technologies and health in low income countries: The potential and the constraints. *Bulletin of the World Health Organization, 79*(9), 850–855.

Charnovitz, S. (2000). The supervision of health and biosafety regulation by world trade rules. *Tulane Environmental Law Journal, 13*, 271–302.

Chatterjee, P. (2004). *The politics of the governed: Reflections on popular politics in most of the world*. New York: Columbia University Press.

Chaudhuri, S., Goldberg, P., & Panle, J. (2003). Estimating the effects of global patent protection in pharmaceuticals: A case study of Quinolones in India. NBER Working Paper 10159. Cambridge, MA: National Bureau of Economic Research.

Chiang, W. Y., & Duann, R. F. (2007). Conceptual metaphors for SARS: "War" between whom? *Discourse & Society, 18*(5), 579–602.

Chitnis, K. (2012). Risk communication and emerging infectious diseases: Lessons and implications for theory-praxis from Avian influenza control. In R. Obregon & S. Waisbord (Eds.), *The Handbook of Global Health Communication* (pp. 408–425). Malden, MA: Wiley-Blackwell.

Christian Aid. (2005). *The economics of failure: The real cost of 'free' trade for poor countries*. London: Christian Aid.

Clapp, J. (2012). *Food*. London: Polity.

Clinton Foundation. (n.d.). Clinton climate initiative. Retrieved from www.clintonfoundation.org/our-work/clinton-climate-initiative on June 1, 2014.

Cockburn, A. (1998). *Whiteout: The CIA, drugs, and the press*. London: Verso.

Cockett, R. (1995). *Thinking the unthinkable: Think tanks and the economic counter-revolution*. London: HarperCollins.

Colas, A. (2005). Neoliberalism, globalization and international relations. In D. Johnston & A. Saad-Filho (Eds.), *Neoliberalism: A critical reader* (pp. 70–80). London: Pluto Press.

Commission on Social Determinants of Health. (2008). *Closing the gap in a generation: Health equity through action on the social determinants of health*. Geneva: World Health Organization.

Connell, R. (2010). Understanding neoliberalism. In S. Braedley & M. Luxton (Eds.), *Neoliberalism and everyday life* (pp. 22–36). Montreal: McGill-Queen's University Press.

Connelly, M. (2008). Fatal misconception: The struggle to control world population. Cambridge: Harvard University Press.

Corman, S. R., Hess, A., & Justus, Z. S. (2006). Credibility in the global war on terrorism: Strategic principles and research agenda. *Consortium for Strategic Communication.* Arizona State University. Report No. 0603, June 9, 2006.

Cornia, G. A. (2001). Globalization and health: Results and options. *Bulletin of the World Health Organization, 79*(9), 834–841.

Croddy, E. C., Hart, C., & Perez-Armendariz, J. (2002). *Chemical and biological warfare.* New York: Springer.

Crouch, C. (2011). *The strange non-death of neoliberalism.* London: Polity.

Cullather, N. (2010). *The hungry world: America's cold war battle against poverty in Asia.* Cambridge, MA: Harvard University Press.

Deering, J., & Singhal, A. (2006). Communication of innovations: A journey with Ev Rogers. In A. Singhal & J. Deering (Eds.), *Communication of innovations: A journey with Ev Rogers* (pp. 15–28). Thousand Oaks, CA: Sage.

Doar, R. (2014). Ten welfare-reform lessons. *National Review.* Retrieved from www.aei.org/article/economics/ten-welfare-reform-lessons/ on April 29, 2014.

Doyle, C., & Patel, P. (2008). Civil society organisations and global health initiatives: Problems of legitimacy. *Social Science & Medicine, 66*(9), 1928–1938.

Dumenil, G., & Levy, D. (2005). The neoliberal (counter-)revolution. In A. Saad-Filho & D. Johnston (Eds.), *Neoliberalism: A critical reader* (pp. 9–19). London: Pluto Press.

Dutta, M. J. (2004a). Poverty, structural barriers, and health: A Santali narrative of health communication. *Qualitative Health Research, 14*(8), 1107–1122.

Dutta, M. J. (2004b). Health attitudes, health cognitions, and health behaviors among Internet health information seekers: Population-based survey. *Journal of Medical Internet Research, 6*(2), 15.

Dutta, M. J. (2006). Theoretical approaches to entertainment education campaigns: A subaltern critique. *Health Communication, 20,* 221–231.

Dutta, M. J. (2007). Communicating about culture and health: Theorizing culture-centered and cultural sensitivity approaches. *Communication Theory, 17*(3), 304–328.

Dutta, M. J. (2008). *Communicating health: A culture-centered approach.* London: Polity.

Dutta, M. J. (2011). *Communicating social change: Structure, culture, agency.* New York: Routledge.

Dutta, M. J. (2013a). Public relations in a global world: Culturally centering theory and praxis. *Asia Pacific Public Relations Journal, 14*(1-2), 21–31.

Dutta, M. J. (2013b). *Voices of resistance.* West Lafayette, IN: Purdue University Press.

Dutta, M. J., & Acharya, L. (2014). Power, control, and the margins in an HIV/AIDS intervention: A culture-centered interrogation of the "Avahan" campaign targeting Indian truckers. *Communication, Culture & Critique.* DOI: 10.1111/cccr.12078

Dutta, M. J., & Basnyat, I. (2008). The Radio Communication Project in Nepal: A culture-centered approach to participation. *Health Education & Behavior, 35*(4), 442–454.

Dutta, M., & Pal, M. (2010). Dialog theory in marginalized settings: A subaltern studies approach. *Communication Theory, 20*(4), 363–386.

Dutta-Bergman, M. J. (2005). Theory and practice in health communication campaigns: A critical interrogation. *Health Communication, 18*(2), 103–122.

Evans, W., Longfield, K., Shekhar, N., Rabemanatsoa, A., Reerink, I., and Snider, J. (2012). Social marketing and condom promotion in Madagascar: A case study in brand equity research. In R. Obregon & S. Waisbord (Eds.), *The Handbook of global health communication* (pp. 330–347). Malden, MA: Wiley-Blackwell.

Everts, J. (2013). Announcing swine flu and the interpretation of pandemic anxiety. *Antipode, 45*(4), 809–825.

Farmer, P. (2001). *Infections and inequalities: The modern plagues.* Berkeley: University of California Press.

Farsetta, D. (2010). Public relations and advertising. In W. H. Wiist (Ed.), *The bottom line or public health: Tactics corporations use to influence health and health policy and what we can do to counter them* (pp. 115–138). Oxford: Oxford University Press.

Faubion, T., Paige, S. B., & Pearson, A. L. (2011). Co-opting the Global Health Agenda: The Problematic Role of Partnerships and Foundations. In S. Rushton & O. D. Willams (Eds.), *Partnerships and foundations in global health governance* (pp. 209–227). New York: Palgrave Macmillan.

Federoff, N. (2011). Engineering food for all. *New York Times*, August 18. Retrieved from www.nytimes.com/2011/08/19/opinion/genetically-engineered-food-for-all.html?_r=0 on July 22, 2014.

Fikree, F. (2005). Reproductive health: A communication challenge in the twenty-first century. In M. Haider (Ed.), *Global public health communication: Challenges, perspectives and strategies* (pp. 173–180). Sudbury, MA: Jones and Bartlett.

Flock, E. (2009). How Bill Gates blew $258 million in India's HIV corridor. *Forbes India*. Retrieved from http://forbesindia.com/article/cross-border/how-bill-gates-blew-$258-million-in-indias-hiv-corridor/852/0 on May 1, 2014.

Forte, M. (2014). Civil society, NGOs, and saving the needy: Imperial neoliberalism. Retrieved from wrongkindofgreen.org/2014/09/01/civil-society-ngos-and-saving-the-needy-imperial-neoliberalism/ on October 11, 2014.

Fourcade-Gourinchas, M., & Babb, S. (2002). The rebirth of the liberal creed: Neoliberalism in four countries. *American Journal of Sociology, 108*, 533–579.

Franks, A. (2005). *Margaret Sanger's eugenic legacy: The control of female fertility.* Jefferson, NC: McFarland.

Gallaher, W. R. (2009). Towards a sane and rational approach to management of Influenza H1N1 2009. *Virology journal, 6*(1), 51.

Garrett, L. (1996). The return of infectious disease. *Foreign Affairs, 75*, 66–79.

Gates Foundation. (2012). *New approaches to the interrogation of anti-malarial compounds.* Retrieved from www.grandchallenges.org/Explorations/Topics/Pages/AntimalarialCompoundsRound9.aspx on June 4, 2014.

Gates Foundation. (2013a). *Develop the next generation of condom: Grand challenges explorations round 11.* Retrieved from www.grandchallenges.org/Explorations/Topics/Pages/NextGenerationCondomRound11.aspx on May 1, 2014.

Gates Foundation. (2013b). *Reinventing the condom.* Retrieved from www.impatientoptimists.org/Posts/2013/03/Reinventing-The-Condom on June 1, 2014.

GATT. (1991). *Thailand restrictions on importation of and internal taxes on cigarettes.* GATT.

George, S. (1997). How to win the war of ideas: Lessons from the Gramscian right. *Dissent, 44*(3), 47–53.

Gershman, J., & Irwin, A. (2000). Getting a grip on the global economy. In J. Y. Kim, J. V. Millen, A. Irwin & J. Gershman (Eds.), *Dying for growth: Global inequality and the health of the poor* (pp. 11–43). Monroe, ME: Common Courage Press.

Gill, A., & Singh, L. (2006). Farmers' suicides and response of public policy: Evidence, diagnosis and alternatives from Punjab. *Economic and Political Weekly*, 2762–2768.

Giroux, Henry A. (2006) *Beyond the spectacle of terrorism: Global uncertainty and the challenge of the new media.* Boulder CO: Paradigm Publishers.

Glasgow, R. E., Bull, S. S., Piette, J. D., & Steiner, J. F. (2004). Interactive behavior change technology: A partial solution to the competing demands of primary care. *American journal of preventive medicine, 27*(2), 80–87.

Goldberg, D. T. (2009). *The threat of race: Reflections on racial neoliberalism.* Malden, MA: Blackwell.

Gordon, D. (2000). The global infectious disease threat and its implications for the United States. Report prepared for the National Intelligence Council. Washington DC: NIC. Retrieved from http://www.fas.org/irp/nic/infectious_diseases_paper.html on February 24, 2015.

Gostin, L. O. (2009). Influenza A (H1N1) and pandemic preparedness under the rule of international law. *JAMA, 301*(22), 2376–2378.

Gourevitch, P. (1984). Breaking with orthodoxy: The politics of economic policy responses to the depression of the 1930s. *International Organization, 38*, 95–129.

Gowan, P. (1999). *The global gamble: Washington's Faustian bid for world dominance.* London: Verso.

Guardian. (2014). Rana plaza: The price of indifference. April 23. Retrieved from www.theguardian.com/commentisfree/2014/apr/23/rana-plaza-price-of-indifference on July 30, 2014.

Guvenen, O. (2013). 2008–2011 world economic crisis, new paradigms, science methodology, information systems, and decision systems. In A. S. Koyuncugil & N. Ozgulbas (Eds.), *Technology and financial crisis: Economical and analytical views* (pp. 1–7). Hershey, PA: IGI Global.

Hall, S. (2003). New Labour's double shuffle. *Soundings, 24*, 10–24.

Hammond, R. (1998). Consolidation in the tobacco industry. *Tobacco Control, 7*(4), 426–428.

Harding, A. (2009). Partnerships with the Private Sector in Health. Washington, DC: Center for Global Development.

Harris, L. M., Baur, C., Donaldson, M., Lefebvre, R., Dugan, E., & Arayasirikul, S. (2013). Health communication and health information technology. In T. Thompson, R. Parrott, & J. Nussbaum (Eds.), *The Routledge handbook of health communication* (pp. 482–497). New York: Routledge.

Hartmann, B. (1995a). Dangerous intersections. *Political Environments, #2*. Retrieved from www.cwpe.org/node/69 on June 20, 2011.

Hartmann, B. (1995b). *Reproductive rights and wrongs: The global politics of population control, revised edition.* Boston: South End Press.

Hartnett, S. J. (2008). The annihilating public policies of the prison-industrial complex; or, crime, violence, and punishment in an age of neoliberalism. *Rhetoric & Public Affairs, 11*(3), 491–515.

Harvey, D. (2001). City and justice: Social movements in the city. In D. Harvey (Ed.), *Spaces of capital: Towards a critical geography* (pp. 188–207). London: Routledge.

Harvey, D. (2003). *The new imperialism.* Oxford: Oxford University Press.

Harvey, D. (2005). *A brief history of neoliberalism.* London: Oxford University Press.

Harvey, D. (2006). *Spaces of global capitalism.* London: Verso.

Hastings, G., Stead, M., McDermott, L., Forsyth, A., MacKintosh, A. M., & Rayner, M. (2006). *Review of research on the effects of food promotion to children. Final report prepared for the Food Standards Agency.* Glasgow: Food Standards Agency Online.

Hawkes, C., Chopra, M., & Friel, S. (2009). Globalization, trade, and the nutrition transition. In Labonté R., Schrecker T., Packer C., & Runnels V. (Eds.), *Globalization and health: Pathways, evidence and policy,* (pp. 235–262). New York: Routledge.

Health Communication Capacity Collaborative. (n.d.). *Demand generation I-Kit for underutilized, life-saving commodities*. Retrieved from sbccimplementationkits.org/demandrmnch/ikitresources/spotlights/ on October 25, 2014.

Healy, D. (2007). The engineers of human souls & academia. *Epidemiologia e psichiatria sociale*, *16*(03), 205–211.

Heinsman, R. (2011). *Workers, unions and global capitalism*. New Delhi: Tulika Books.

Hewlett, B. S., & Amola, R. P. (2003). Cultural contexts of Ebola in northern Uganda. *Emerging infectious diseases*, *9*(10), 1242.

Holt-Gimenez, E., & Patel, R. (2009). *Food rebellion: Crisis and the hunger for justice*. Oakland, CA: Food First Books.

Horn, D. (2013). Locating security in the womb: U.S. foreign policy, population control and international family planning programs. *International Feminist Journal of Politics*, *15*, 195–212.

Hornik, R. (1973). *Mass media participation and modernization: A causal analysis*. PhD diss., Stanford University.

Human Terrain System. (n.d.). *Human terrain system*. Retrieved from humanterrainsystem.army.mil/ on June 24, 2014.

Hyatt, R. R. (2007). Military spending: Global health threat or global public good. In I. Kawachi & S. Wamala (Eds.), *Globalization and health* (pp. 311–330). Oxford: Oxford University Press.

Ibrahim, Y. (2007). SARS and the rhetoric of war in Singapore. *Crossroads: An Interdisciplinary Journal of Southeast Asian Studies*, *18*(2), 90–119.

Ibrahim, S., & Hulme, D. (2011). Civil society and poverty. In M. Edwards (Ed.), *The Oxford handbook of civil society* (pp. 391–403). Oxford: Oxford University Press.

Institute of Medicine (US). Committee on Communication for Behavior Change in the 21st Century, & Improving the Health of Diverse Populations. (2002). *Speaking of health: Assessing health communication strategies for diverse populations*. Washington, DC: Joseph Henry Press.

International Consortium of Investigative Journalists (ICIJ). (2015). Banking giant HSBC sheltered murky cash linked to dictators and arms dealers. Retrieved from http://www.icij.org/project/swiss-leaks/banking-giant-hsbc-sheltered-murky-cash-linked-dictators-and-arms-dealers on February 9, 2015.

Kaldor, M. (2003). *Global civil society: An answer to war*. Cambridge: Polity Press.

Kamat, S. (2004). The privatization of public interest: Theorizing NGO discourse in a neoliberal era. *Review of International Political Economy*, *11*(1), 155–76.

Kapilashrami, A., & O'Brien, O. (2012). The Global Fund and the re-configuration and re-emergence of "civil society": Widening or closing the democratic deficit? *Global Public Health*, *7*(5), 437–451.

Karim, S. A. (2009). From 'playstation thumb' to 'cellphone thumb': the new epidemic in teenagers. *SAMJ: South African Medical Journal*, *99*(3), 161–162.

Kashefi, E., & Mort, M. (2004). Grounded citizens' juries: A tool for health activism?. *Health Expectations*, *7*(4), 290–302.

Keil, R., & Ali, S. H. (2008). "Racism is a weapon of mass destruction": SARS and the social fabric of urban multiculturalism. *Networked Disease: Emerging Infections in the Global City*, *55*, 152–166.

Kesavachandran, C., Rastogi, S. K., Das, M., & Khan, A. M. (2006). Working conditions and health among employees at information technology-enabled services: A review of current evidence. *Indian Journal of Medical Sciences, 7*, 300–307. Retrieved from www.bioline.org.br/request?ms06044 on June 2, 2014.

Kim, Y. M., et al. (1992). Improving the quality of service delivery in Nigeria. *Studies in Family Planning, 23*, 118–127.

Kimura, A. H. (2013). *Hidden hunger: Gender and the politics of smarter foods*. Ithaca, NY: Cornell University Press.

King, N. B. (2002). Security, disease, commerce ideologies of postcolonial global health. *Social Studies of Science, 32*(5–6), 763–789.

King, S. (2006). *Pink Ribbons Inc.: Breast cancer and the politics of philanthropy*. Minneapolis: University of Minnesota Press.

Koblentz, G. D. (2010). Biosecurity reconsidered: Calibrating biological threats and responses. *International Security, 34*(4), 96–132.

Kreps, G., Alibek, K., Neuhauser, L., Rowan, K., & Sparks, L. (2005). Emergency/risk communication to promote public health and biological threats. In M. Haider (Ed.), *Global public health communication: Challenges, perspectives, and strategies* (pp. 349–362). Sudbury, MA: Jones and Bartlett Publishers.

Kreuter, M. W., Farrell, D. W., Olevitch, L. R., & Brennan, L. K. (2013). *Tailoring health messages: Customizing communication with computer technology*. New York: Routledge.

Kumar, S., & Butler, D. (2013). Calls in India for action against U.S. charity. *Nature*. Retrieved from www.nature.com/news/calls-in-india-for-legal-action-against-us-charity-1.13700 on June 18, 2014.

Labonté, R. (2009). The global financial crisis and health: Scaling up our effort. *Canadian Journal of Public Health/Revue Canadienne de Santeѐ Publique, 100*, 173–175.

Labonté, R., & Schrecker, T. (2007). Globalization and social determinants of health: The role of the global marketplace (part 2 of 3). *Globalization and Health, 3*(6), 1–17.

Labonté, R., Schrecker, T., Packer, C., & Runnels, V. (Eds.). (2010). *Globalization and health: Pathways, evidence and policy*. New York: Routledge.

Lane, R. (2013). The thinker and the salesman: Bill Gates and Bono on solving global poverty. *Forbes India*. Retrieved from forbesindia.com/article/cross-border/the-thinker-and-the-salesman-bill-gates-and-bono-on-solving-global-poverty/36627/1?utm=slidebox on June 4, 2014.

Larson, B. M., Nerlich, B., & Wallis, P. (2005). Metaphors and biorisks: The war on infectious diseases and invasive species. *Science Communication, 26*(3), 243–268.

Laurell, A. (2000). Structural adjustment and the globalization of social policy in Latin America. *International Sociology, 15*, 306–25.

Lee, M. (2014). A review of communication scholarship on the financial markets and the financial media. *International Journal of Communication, 8*, 22.

Leigh, L., Ball, J., Garside, J., & Pegg, D. (2015). HSBC files show how Swiss Bank helped clients dodge taxes and hide millions. *The Guardian*. Retrieved from http://www.theguardian.com/business/2015/feb/08/hsbc-files-expose-swiss-bank-clients-dodge-taxes-hide-millions?CMP=share_btn_tw on on February 22, 2015.

Lerner, D. (1958). *The passing of traditional society*. New York: Free Press.

Levine, M., & Kavanau-Levine, L. (1993). *The big white lie: The CIA and the cocaine/crack epidemic*. New York: Thunder's Mouth Press.

Levy, B. S., & Sidel, V. W. (Eds.). (1997). *War and public health*. Oxford: Oxford University Press.

Lewis, S. J., Kaltofen, M., & Ormsby, G. (1991). *Border trouble: Rivers in peril. A report on water pollution due to industrial development in Northern Mexico*. Boston: National Toxics Campaign Fund.

Liagin, E. (1996). Profit or loss: Cooking the books at USAID. *PRI Review*, *6*(3). Retrieved from http://pop.org/content/profit-or-loss-cooking-the-books-at-usaid-1207 on July 10, 2014.

Lin, C. A. (2007). An integrated communication technology and social change typology. In C. Lin & D. Atkin (Eds.), *Communication Technology and Social Change: Theory and Implications*, (pp. 3-16). Mahwah, NJ: Lawrence Erlbaum.

Loevinsohn, B., & Harding, A. (2005). Buying results? Contracting for health service delivery in developing countries. *Lancet*, *366*(9486), 676–681.

London, L., & Schneider, H. (2012). Globalisation and health inequalities: Can a human rights paradigm create space for civil society action? *Social Science & Medicine*, *74*(1), 6–13.

Loriaux, M. M. (1997). *Capital ungoverned: liberalizing finance in interventionist states*. Ithaca, NY: Cornell University Press.

Loyd, J. (2009). "A microscopic insurgent": Militarization, health, and critical geographies of violence. *Annals of the Association of American Geographers*, *99*(5), 863–873.

Lupton, D. (1994). Toward the development of critical health communication praxis. *Health Communication*, *6*(1), 55–67.

Lupton, D. (1995). *The imperative of health: Public health and the regulated body*. London: Sage.

Malthus, T. R. (1966). *First essay on population, 1798* (Vol. 14). New York: Macmillan.

Marazzi, C. (2011). *The violence of financial capitalism*. Boston, MA: MIT Press Books.

Marcy, W. L. (2010). *The politics of cocaine: How U.S. foreign policy has created a thriving drug industry in Central and South America*. Chicago: Chicago Review Press.

Marmot, M. (2004). *The status syndrome: How your social standing affects your health and life expectancy*. London: Bloomsbury.

Marmot, M., & Wilkinson, R. (Eds.) (2006). *Social determinants of health*. Oxford: Oxford University Press.

Massoglia, M. (2008). Incarceration, health, and racial disparities in health. *Law and Society Review*, *42*, 172–306.

Mazzarella, W. (2010). Beautiful balloon: The digital divide and the charisma on new media in India. *American Ethnologist*, *37*, 783–804.

McCoy, D., Chand, S., & Sridhar, D. (2009). Global health funding: How much, where it comes from and where it goes. *Health Policy Plan*, 24, 407–417.

McCoy, D., & McGoey, L. (2011). Global health and the Gates Foundation—in perspective. In S. Rushton & O. D. Williams (Eds.), *Partnerships and foundations in global health governance* (pp. 143–163). New York: Palgrave MacMillan.

Melkote, S. R., & Steeves, H. L. (2001). *Communication for development in the Third World: Theory and practice for empowerment*. London: Sage.

Michaelis, M., Doerr, H. W., & Cinatl Jr, J. (2009). Novel swine-origin influenza A virus in humans: Another pandemic knocking at the door. *Medical microbiology and immunology*, *198*(3), 175–183.

Millen, J., & Holtz, T. (2000). Dying for growth, part I: Transnational corporations and the health of the poor. In J. Y. Kim, J. V. Millen, A. Irwin, & J. Gershman (Eds.), *Dying for growth: Global inequality and the health of the poor* (pp. 177–223). Monroe, ME: Common Courage Press.

Millen, J., Irwin, A., & Kim, J. (2000). Introduction: What is growing? Who is dying? In J. Y. Kim, J. V. Millen, A. Irwin, & J. Gershman (Eds.), *Dying for growth: Global inequality and the health of the poor* (pp. 3–10). Monroe, ME: Common Courage Press.

Mirchandani, K. (2004). Practices of global capital: Gaps, cracks and ironies in transnational call centers in India. *Global Networks*, *4*, 355–374.

Mirowski, P., & Plehwe, D. (Eds.). (2009). *The road from Mont Pelerin*. Cambridge, MA: Harvard University Press.

Monahan, T. (2010). *Surveillance in the time of insecurity*. New Brunswick, NJ: Rutgers University Press.

Monteiro, C., Conde, W., & Popkin, B. (2004). Obesity and inequities in health in the developing world. *International Journal of Obesity*, *28*, 1181–1186.

Moreton, B. (2009). *To serve God and Wal-Mart: The making of Christian free enterprise*. Cambridge, MA: Harvard University Press.

Mosher, S. W. (2008). *Population control: Real costs, illusory benefits*. New Brunswick, NJ: Transaction Publishers.

Muhammad, A. (2009). Grameen and Microcredit: a tale of corporate success. *Economic and Political Weekly*, *xliv*(35), 35–42.

Münster, D., & Münster, U. (2012). Consuming the forest in an environment of crisis: Nature tourism, forest conservation and neoliberal agriculture in South India. *Development and Change*, *43*(1), 205–227.

Muntaner, C., Salazar, R. M., Benach, J., & Armada, F. (2006). Venezuela's barrio adentro: An alternative to neoliberalism in health care. *International Journal of Health Services*, *36*, 803–811.

Murphy, E., & Gryboski, K. (2005). The importance of client–provider interactions: Evidence from family planning programs. In M. Haider (Ed.), *Global public health communication: Challenges, perspectives, and strategies* (pp. 199–216). Sudbury, MA: Jones & Bartlett Publishers.

Narayan, D. (Ed.). (2000). *Can anyone hear us?* (Vol. 1). New York: World Bank Publications.

Narayan, D., Patel, R., Schafft, K., Rademacher, A., & Koch-Schulte, S. (1999a). *Dying for change: Poor people's experience of health and ill-health*. Washington, DC: World Bank.

Narayan, D., Patel, R., Schafft, K., Rademacher, A., & Koch-Schulte, S. (1999b). *Voices of the poor: Can anyone hear us?* Washington, DC: World Bank.

Narayan, D., & Petesch, P. (2002). *Voices of the poor: From many lands*. Washington, DC: World Bank.

National Association of Professional Environmentalists. (2012). *A study on land grabbing cases in Uganda*. Kampala, Uganda: Author.

Navarro, V. (2007). *Neoliberalism, globalization, and inequalities: Consequences for health and quality of life*. Amityville, NY: Baywood.

Nayak, P. K., & Berkes, F. (2008). Politics of co-optation: Community forest management versus joint forest management in Orissa, India. *Environmental Management*, *41*(5), 707–718.

Ndiaye, K. (2014). Highlighting the C in ICT: Key communication and culture questions in ICT for health. *Journal of Health Communication*, *19*(5), 529–531.

Nestle, M. (2013). *Food politics: How the food industry influences nutrition and health*. Vol. 3. Berkeley: University of California Press.

Nordenstreng, K. (2012). The history of NWICO and its lessons. In *From NWICO to WSIS: 30 years of communication geopolitics. Actors and flows, structures and divides* (pp. 29—40). Bristol: Intellect Ltd.

Nordstrom, C. (2007). *Global outlaws: crime, money, and power in the contemporary world*. Berkeley: University of California Press.

Obi, C. I. (1997). Globalisation and local resistance: The case of the Ogoni versus Shell. *New Political Economy*, *2*(1), 137–148.

Olivera, O., & Lewis, T. (2004). *Cochabamba!: Water war in Bolivia*. Cambridge, MA: South End Press.

Oreskes, N., & Conway, E. (2010). *Merchants of doubt: How a handful of scientists obscured the truth on issues from tobacco smoke to global warming*. New York: Bloomsbury Press.

Padel, F., & Das, S. (2010). *Out of this earth: East India adivasis and the aluminium cartel*. Hyderabad, India: Orient Blackswan.

Panitch, L., & Gindin, S. (2004). Global capitalism and American empire. *Socialist Register, 40,* 12–28.

Panitch, L., & Gindin, S. (2005). Global finance and American empire. *Social Register, 41,* 43–52.

Panitch, L., & Konings, M. (2009). Myths of neoliberal deregulation. *New Left Review, 57*(May/June), 67–83.

PATH. (n.d). PATH's guiding principle for private sector collaboration. Retrieved from www.path.org/publications/files/ER_gp_collab.pdf on June 18, 2014.

Pavarala, V., & Malik, K. K. (2007). *Other voices: The struggle for community radio in India*. New Delhi: Sage.

Peck, J. (2001). Neoliberalizing states: thin policies/hard outcomes. *Progress in Human Geography*, *25*(3), 445–455.

Peck, J., & Tickell, A. (2002). Neoliberalizing space. *Antipode*, *34*(3), 380–404.

Peet, R. (2003). *Unholy trinity: The IMF, the World Bank, and the WTO*. London: Zed Books.

Petras, J. (1997). Imperialism and NGOs in Latin America. *Monthly Review, 49*. Retrieved from monthlyreview.org/1997/12/01/imperialism-and-ngos-in-latin-america on October 31, 2013.

Petras, J. (1999). NGOs: In the service of imperialism. *Journal of Contemporary Asia*, *29*(4), 429–440.

Pfeiffer, J. (2003). International NGOs and primary health care in Mozambique: The need for a new model of collaboration. *Social Science & Medicine*, *56*(4), 725–738.

Pfeiffer, J., & Chapman, R. (2010). Anthropological perspectives on structural adjustment and public health. *Annual Review of Anthropology*, *39*, 149–165.

Phelps, B. (2012). Opinion: Biofortification is an obstacle to food justice. Retrieved from www.freshfruitportal.com/2012/09/12/opinion-biofortification-is-an-obstacle-to-food-justice/?country=singapore on October 29, 2013.

Pickard, V. (2007). Neoliberal visions and revisions in global communications policy from NWICO to WSIS. *Journal of Communication Inquiry*, *31*(2), 118–139.

Piketty, T. (2014). *Capital in the 21st century*. Cambridge, MA: Harvard University Press.

Piotrow, P. T., Kincaid, D. L., Rimon, J. G., Rinehart, W., & Samson, K. (1997). *Health communication: lessons from family planning and reproductive health*. Westport, CT: Prager.

Piotrow, P. T., Treiman, K. A., Rimon, J. G., Yun, S. H., & Lozare, B. V. (1994). Strategies for family planning promotion. Washington, DC: World Bank.

Plehwe, D. (2008). Im Schatten von Hayek und Friedman: Die Vielflieger im Kreise der Mont Pèlerin Society. *Transnationale Netzwerke im, 20*, 235–264.

Plehwe, D. (2013). Think tanks in America. *Critical Policy Studies, 7*(4), 471–474.

Plehwe, D., Walpen, B. J., & Neunhöffer, G. (Eds.). (2007). *Neoliberal hegemony: A global critique*. New York: Routledge.

Poole. I. (1982). *Technologies of freedom*. Cambridge, MA: MIT Press.

Powell, F. (2007). *The politics of civil society: Neoliberalism or social left*. Bristol: Policy Press.

Powell, L. M., Harris, J. L., & Fox, T. (2013). Food marketing expenditures aimed at youth: Putting the numbers in context. *American Journal of Preventive Medicine, 45*, 453–461.

Prasad, M. (2006). *The politics of free markets: The rise of neoliberal economic policies in Britain, France, Germany, and the United States*. Chicago: University of Chicago Press.

Pun, N. (2005a). Global production, company codes of conduct, and labor conditions in China: A case study of two factories. *China Journal, 54*, 101–113.

Pun, N. (2005b). *Made in China: Women factory workers in a global workplace*. Durham, NC: Duke University Press.

Pun, N., & Chan J. W. (2004). Community based labor organizing. *International Union Rights, 11*(4), 10–11.

Pun, N., & Smith, C. (2005). *Putting transnational labour process in its place: Dormitory labour regime in post-socialist China*. Paper presented at the 22nd International Labour Process Conference, April 5–7, Amsterdam.

Pyagbara, L. S. (2007). The adverse impacts of oil pollution on the environment and wellbeing of a local indigenous community: The experience of the Ogoni people of Nigeria. In *International Expert Group meeting on indigenous peoples and protection of the environment*. Retrieved from www.un.org/esa/socdev/unpfii/documents/workshop_IPPE_pyagbara on May 30, 2012.

Qiu, J. L. (2012). Network labour: Beyond the shadow of Foxconn. In L. Hjorth, J. Burgess, & I. Richardson (Eds.), *Studying mobile media: Cultural technologies, mobile communication, and the iPhone* (pp. 173–189). New York: Routledge.

Rajan, K. S. (2006). *Biocapital: The constitution of postgenomic life*. Durham, NC: Duke University Press.

Ramon, S. (2008). Neoliberalism and its implications for mental health in the UK. *International Journal of Law and Psychiatry, 31*(2), 116–125.

Rampton, S., & Stauber, J. (2001). *Trust us, we're experts*. New York: Putnam.

Rauch, J. (2007). This is not charity. *Atlantic*, October, 64–76.

Ravishankar, N., Gubbin, P., Cooley, R., Leach-Kemon, K., Michaud, C., Jamison, D., & Murray, C. (2009). Financing global health: Tracking development assistance for health from 1990 to 2007. *Lancet, 373*, 2113–2124.

Richardson, J., & Harris, J. (2011). Food marketing and social media. American University Digital Food Marketing Conference.

Rostow, W. W. (1960). *The stages of growth: A non-communist manifesto*. Cambridge: Cambridge University Press.

Renganathan, E., Hosein, E., Parks, W., Lloyd, L., Suhaili, M. R., & Odugleh, A. (2005). Communication-for-behavioral-impact (COMBI): A review of WHO's experiences with strategic social mobilization and communication in the prevention and control of communicable diseases. In M. Haider (Ed.), *Global public health communication: Challenges, perspectives, and strategies* (pp. 305–320). Sudbury, MA: Jones and Bartlett Publishing.

Robinson, W. I. (1996a). Globalization, the world system, and "democracy promotion" in U.S. foreign policy. *Theory and Society*, *25*, 615–665.

Robinson, W. I. (1996b). *Promoting polyarchy: Globalization, U.S. intervention, and hegemony*. Cambridge: Cambridge University Press.

Robinson, W. I. (2004). *A theory of global capitalism: Production, class, and state in a transnational world*. Baltimore: Johns Hopkins University Press.

Rodgers, Daniel T. (2001). *The revival of market ideology*. Unpublished manuscript, Princeton University.

Rogers, E. M. (1962). *Diffusion of innovations*. New York: Free Press.

Rogers, E. M. (1971). *Social change in rural society*. Englewood Cliffs, NJ: Prentice Hall.

Rogers, E. M. (1973). *Communication strategies for family planning*. New York: Free Press.

Rogers, E. M. (1974). Communication in development. *Annals of the American Academy of Political and Social Science*, *412*, 44–54.

Rogers, E. M. (1983). *Diffusion of innovations*. New York: Free Press.

Rogers, E. M. (1995). *Diffusion of innovations*. New York: Free Press.

Rogers, E. M. (2003). *Diffusion of innovations*. New York: Free Press.

Rogers, E. M., & Svenning, L. (1969). *Modernization among peasants: The impact of communication*. New York: Holt, Rinehart & Winston.

Rose, N. (2001). The politics of life itself. *Theory, Culture & Society*, *18*(6), 1–30.

Rose, N. (2007). *The politics of life itself*. Princeton, NJ: Princeton University Press.

Rowden, R. (2009). *The deadly ideas of neoliberalism: How the IMF has undermined public health and the fight against AIDS*. New York: Zed Books.

Ryan, B., & Gross, N. C. (1943). The diffusion of hybrid seed corn in two Iowa communities. *Rural sociology*, *8*(1), 15–24.

Saad-Filho, A., & Johnston, D. (2005). Introduction. In A. Saad-Filho & D. Johnston (Eds.), *Neoliberalism: A critical reader*. London: Pluto Press.

Salinsky, E. (2002, April). Public Health Emergency Preparedness: Fundamentals of the "System". National Health Policy Forum.

Samara, T. R. (2010). Order and security in the city: Producing race and policing neoliberal spaces in South Africa. *Ethnic and Racial Studies*, *33*(4), 637–655.

Sastry, S., & Dutta, M. J. (2012). Public health, global surveillance, and the "emerging disease" worldview: A postcolonial appraisal of PEPFAR. *Health Communication*, *27*(6), 519–532.

Scherer, F. M. (2004). A note on global welfare in pharmaceutical patenting. *World Economics*, *27*, 1127–1128.

Schoepf, B. G., Schoepf, C., & Millen, J. V. (2000). Theoretical therapies, remote remedies: SAPs and the political ecology of health in Africa. In J. Y. Kim, J. V. Millen, A. Irwin, & J. Gershman (Eds.), *Dying for growth: Global inequality and the health of the poor* (pp. 91–125). Monroe, ME: Common Courage Press.

Schuller, M. (2009). Gluing globalization: NGOs as intermediaries in Haiti. *PoLAR: Political and Legal Anthropology Review*, *32*(1), 84–104.

Shadlen, K. C. (2007). The political economy of AIDS treatment: Intellectual property and the transformation of generic supply. *International Studies Quarterly*, *51*, 559–581.

Shah, H. (2011). *The production of modernization: Daniel Lerner, mass media, and the passing of traditional society*. Philadelphia: Temple University Press.

Shermer, M. (2013). The liberal's war on science. *Scientific American*, January 15. Retrieved from www.scientificamerican.com/article/the-liberals-war-on-science/ on June 10, 2014.

Shiva, V. (1988). Reductionist science as epistemic violence. In A. Nandy (Ed.), *Science, hegemony, and violence* (pp. 157–184). New Delhi: Oxford University Press.

Shiva, V. (1989). *Staying alive: Women, ecology, and development*. London: Zed.

Shiva, V. (1991). *The violence of the green revolution: Third World agriculture, ecology and politics*. London: Zed.

Shiva, V. (2000). *Stolen harvest: The hijacking of the global food supply*. Cambridge, MA: South End Press.

Shiva, V. (2001). Democratizing biology: Reinventing biology from a feminist, ecological, and Third World perspective. In M. Lederman & I. Bartsch (Eds.), *The gender and science reader* (pp. 447–465). London: Routledge.

Shiva, V. (2002). Seeds of suicide: The ecological and human cost of globalization of agriculture. In V. Shiva & G. Bedi (Eds.), *Sustainable agriculture and food security: The impact of globalization* (pp. 169–183). New Delhi: Sage.

Shiva, V. (2005). *Earth democracy: Justice, sustainability and peace*. Cambridge, MA: South End Press.

Shiva, V. (2007). *Wheat biopiracy: The real issues the government is avoiding*. Retrieved from www.zcommunications.org/wheat-biopiracy-the-real-issues-the-government-is-avoiding-by-vandana2–shiva.pdf on May 15, 2010.

Shiva, V. (2010). Press statement on Bt. Brinjal and GM foods. January 12. Retrieved from www.navdanya.org/news/81–press-statement-on-bt-brinjal-a-gm-foods on March 1, 2010.

Shiva, V., Anderson, P., Schücking, H., Gray, A., Lohmann, L., & Cooper, D. (1991). *Biodiversity: Social and ecological perspectives*. London: Zed.

Shiva, V., & Bedi, G. (2002). *Sustainable agriculture and food security: The impact of globalization*. New Delhi: Sage.

Shiva, V., & Jafri, A. H. (2003). *Failure of the GMOs in India*. Retrieved from www.mindfully.org/GE/2003/India-GMO-Failure-Shiva31may03.htm on March 1, 2010.

Shiva, V., Jafri, A. H., Emani, A., & Pande, M. (2002). *Seeds of suicide: The ecological and human costs of globalization stone, biotechnology and suicide in India of agriculture* (Rev. ed.). New Delhi: Research Foundation for Science, Technology and Ecology.

Shome, R. (2006). Thinking through the diaspora: Call centers, India, and a new politics or hybridity. *International Journal of Cultural Studies*, *9*, 105–124

Shugart, H. A. (2010). Consuming citizen: Neoliberating the obese body. *Communication, Culture, and Critique*, *3*, 105–126.

Slezak, T., et al. (2003). Comparative genomics tools applied to bioterrorism defense. *Briefings in Bioinformatics*, *4*, 133–149.

Smith, R. (2005). In M. Haider (Ed.), *Global public health communication: Challenges, perspectives, and strategies* (pp. 199–216). Sudbury, MA: Jones & Bartlett Publishers.

Smith, R. A., Witte, K., & Lazell, C. K. (2005). Social change interventions in public health communication. In M Haider and R. Pal (Eds.), *Global public health communication: Challenges, perspectives and strategies* (pp. 59–65). Sudbury, MA: Jones and Bartlett Publishers.

Smolinski, M., Hamburg, M., & Lederberg, J. (2003). *Microbial threats to health emergence, detection, and response*. Washington, DC: National Academy Press.

Sow, P., & Ward, S. (2013). Continuing the condom conversation. *Impatient Optimists*. Retrieved from http://www.impatientoptimists.org/Posts/2013/03/Reinventing-The-Condom on August 13, 2014.

Sparke, M. (2009). On denationalization as neoliberalization: Biopolitics, class interest, and the incompleteness of citizenship. *Political Power and Social Theory, 20*, 287–300.

Speidel, J., Sinding, S., Gillespie, D., Maguire, E., & Neuse, M. (2009). *Making the case for U.S. international family planning assistance*. Retrieved from www.jhsph.edu on January 10, 2014.

Sreekumar, T. T. (2011). *ICTS and development in India: Perspectives on the rural network society*. London: Anthem Press.

Stead, M., McDermott, L., Forsyth, A., MacKintosh, A. M., Rayner, M., Godfrey, C., & Angus, K. (2003). *Review of research on the effects of food promotion to children*. Glasgow: Centre for Social Marketing, University of Strathclyde.

Stiegler, B. (2010). *For a new critique of political economy*. London: Polity.

Storey, D., & Figueroa, M. (2012). Toward a global theory of health behavior and social change. In R. Obregon & S. Waisbord (Eds.), *The handbook of global health communication* (pp. 70–93). Malden, MA: Wiley-Blackwell.

Stuckler, D., Basu, S., & McKee, M. (2011). Global health philanthropy and institutional relationships: How should conflicts of interest be addressed?. *PLoS Medicine, 8*(4), e1001020. doi:10.1371/journal.pmed.1001020

Subramanian, A. (1994). Putting some numbers on the TRIPS pharmaceutical debate. *International Journal of Technology Management, 10*, 1–17.

Sudhashree, V. P., Rohith, K., & Shrinivas, K. (2005). Issues and concerns of health among call center employees. *Indian Journal of Occupational and Environmental Medicine, 9*, 129–132.

Suggs, L. S., & Ratzan, S. C. (2012). Global e-health communication. In R. Obregon & S. Waisbord (Eds.), *The handbook of global health communication* (pp. 251–273). Malden, MA: Wiley-Blackwell.

SumofUs. (n.d.). Unilever: I know what rainforests look like. Retrieved from action.sumofus.org/a/unilever-palm-oil/ on August 20, 2014.

Sunder Rajan, K. (2006). *Biocapital*. Durham, NC: Duke University Press.

Teo, P., Yeoh, B. S., & Ong, S. N. (2005). SARS in Singapore: Surveillance strategies in a globalising city. *Health Policy, 72*(3), 279–291.

Teutsch, S. M., & Churchill, R. E. (Eds.). (2000). *Principles and practice of public health surveillance*. Oxford: Oxford University Press.

Thomas, P. N. (2011). *Negotiating communication rights: Case studies from India*. New Delhi: Sage.

Timmer, A. D. (2010). Constructing the "needy subject": NGO discourses of Roma need. *PoLAR: Political and Legal Anthropology Review, 33*(2), 264–281.

Timmerman, L. (2010). *Steve Davis, the techie turned global healthie, gets dose of reality at close range in India*. Retrieved from www.xconomy.com/seattle/2010/11/05/steve-davis-the-techie-turned-global-healthie-gets-dose-of-reality-at-close-range-in-india/ on August 28, 2014.

Transnational Institute. (2013). *The global land grab: A primer*. Retrieved from www.tni.org/primer/global-land-grab on March 7, 2014.

Tsing, A. L. (2011). *Friction: An ethnography of global connection*. Princeton, NJ: Princeton University Press.

Trade and Environment Database (TED). (1998). Basmati. *TED Case Studies, 8*(2). Retrieved from http://www1.american.edu/ted/TED/all.html on February 23, 2015.

Turshen, M. (1999). *Privatizing health services in Africa*. New Brunswick, NJ: Rutgers University Press.

Unger, J. P., De Paepe, P., Ghilbert, P., Soors, W., & Green, A. (2006). Disintegrated care: The Achilles heel of international health policies in low and middle-income countries. *International Journal of Integrated Care, 6*, 1–13.

United Nations Conference on Trade and Development. (2006). *The least developed countries report 2006: Developing productive capacities*. New York: United Nations Conference on Trade and Development.

Unwin, P. T. H. (Ed.). (2009). *ICT4D: Information and communication technology for development*. Cambridge: Cambridge University Press.

Valente, T. (2011). Social networks and health communication. In T. Thompson, R. Parrott, & J. Nussbaum (Eds.), *The Routledge handbook of health communication* (pp. 519–531). New York: Routledge.

Van der Geest, W., & Van Der Hoeven, R. (Eds.). (1999). *Adjustment, employment & missing institutions in Africa: The experience in Eastern & Southern Africa*. Geneva: International Labour Organization.

Van der Hoeven, R. (2000). *Poverty and structural adjustment: Some remarks on tradeoffs between equity and growth*. Geneva: Employment Sector, International Labour Office.

Vedanta. (2010). *The Lanjigarh development story*. London: Vedanta.

Villar, O. (2007). U.S. narcocolonialism? Colombian cocaine and twenty-first century imperialism. *Research in Political Economy, 24*, 97–128.

Viswanath K. (2011). Cyberinfrastructure: An extraordinary opportunity to bridge health and communication inequalities? *American Journal of Preventive Medicine, 40*(5S2), S245–S248.

Viswanath, K., & Kreuter, M. W. (2007). Health disparities, communication inequalities, and e-health: A commentary. *American Journal of Preventive Medicine, 32*(5), S131.

Vitali, S., Glattfelder,J. B., & Battiston, S. (2011). The network of global corporate control. *PLoS One, 10*, 1–6.

Waitzkin, H. (1991). *The politics of medical encounters*. New Haven, CT: Yale University Press.

Waitzkin, H. (2011). *Medicine and public health at the end of empire*. Boulder, CO: Paradigm Publishers.

Waitzkin, H., & Modell, H. (1974). Medicine, socialism, and totalitarianism: Lessons from Chile. *New England Journal of Medicine, 291*, 171–177.

Ward, K., & England, K. (2007). Introduction: Reading neoliberalization. In K. England & K. Ward (Eds.), *Neoliberalization: States, networks, peoples* (pp. 1–22). Malden, MA: Blackwell Publishing.

Webb, G. (1998). *Dark alliance*. New York: Seven Stories Press.

Weber, M. (1905). *The Protestant ethic and the spirit of capitalism*. New York: Routledge.

Williams, O. D., & Rushton, S. (2011). Private actors in global health governance. In S. Rushton & O. D. Williams (Eds.), *Partnerships and foundations in global health governance* (pp. 1–25). New York: Palgrave Macmillan.

Wilson, M. G., Lavis, J. N., & Guta, A. (2012). Community-based organizations in the health sector: A scoping review. *Health Research Policy and Systems, 10*(36), 10–1186.

Woods, M. (2002). Food for thought: the biopiracy of jasmine and basmati rice. *Albany Law Journal of Science & Technology, 13*, 123.

World Health Organization. (2003). *Severe acute respiratory syndrome: Status of the outbreak and lessons for the immediate future.* Geneva: World Heath Organization. Retrieved from www.who.int/csr/media/sars_wha.pdf on February 24, 2015.

World Health Organization. (2006). *SARS: How a global epidemic was stopped.* Geneva: World Health Organization.

World Health Organization. (2008). *Closing the gap in a generation: Health equity through action on the social determinants of health. Final report of the Commission on Social Determinants of Health.* Geneva: World Health Organization.

World Health Organization. (2014). *What this—the largest Ebola outbreak in history—tells the world.* Retrieved from www.who.int/csr/disease/ebola/ebola-6-months/lessons/en/ on October 21, 2014.

Yach, D, Wipfli, H., Hammond, R., & Glantz, S. (2008). Globalization and tobacco. In I. Kawachi & S. Wamala (Eds.), *Globalization and Health* (pp. 39–67). Oxford: Oxford University Press.

Yale Rudd Center for Food Policy & Obesity. (n.d.) Retrieved from http://www.yalerud-dcenter.org/legislation/search.aspx on February 24, 2015.

Yergin, D., & Stanislaw, J. (1999). *The commanding heights: The battle between government and market place that is remaking the modern world.* New York: Simon and Schuster.

Youde, J. (2011). The Clinton Foundation and global health governance. In S. Rushton & O. D. Williams (Eds.), *Partnerships and foundations in global health governance* (pp. 164–183). New York: Palgrave Macmillan.

Youde, J. (2012). *Global health governance.* London: Polity.

Zoller, H., & Dutta, M. J. (2008). *Emerging perspectives in health communication: Meaning, culture, and power.* New York: Routledge.

INDEX

ABOUT THE AUTHOR

Mohan J. Dutta is Provost's Chair Professor and Head of the Department of Communications and New Media at the National University of Singapore. He is also Joint Professor in the Interactive Digital Media Institute at the National University of Singapore and Adjunct Professor of Communication at the Brian Lamb School of Communication at Purdue University. Dutta is the director of the Center for Culture-Centered Approach to Research and Evaluation at the National University of Singapore. He is one of the most prolific scholars in health communication, author of over 150 journal articles and book chapters, and author or editor of six books. He was recognized in 2006 as the Lewis Donohew Outstanding Scholar in Health Communication and as the Lim Chong Yah Professor of Communications and New Media at the National University of Singapore.